**IMG Friendly Internal Medicine Residency Programs List**

**With Comprehensive Match Selection Criteria and Programs Requirements**

**By**

**IMG Guide**

**And**

**Applicant Guide**

## Table of Contents

# Introduction

# IMG Friendly Internal Medicine Residency Programs List

In Collaboration between the Applicant Guide and the IMG Guide we present to you the most complete and up-to-date IMG friendly internal medicine residency programs list with full match selection criteria and requirements for these programs. This book is essentially written for international medical graduates seeking residency in the US. The idea of writing this book came from our insight that many IMGs every year don't match because they don't know where to apply. Most of the time, they end applying to programs that don't have IMGs or those that don't match their criteria hence they end losing money with no interviews earned. The information was gathered from program directors, coordinators, chiefs, faculty and residents. It includes Programs names, Programs codes, States, Addresses, Phones, Faxes, Percentage of IMGs in the programs, Minimum USMLE Step 1 and Step 2 Score Requirements, Attempts on any step, CS requirement at time of application, USCE Requirements, Cut-Off time since graduation, Programs offering couple match and Visas Sponsored or accepted.

## Alabama

### University of Alabama Medical Center (Huntsville) Internal Medicine Residency Program

**Specialty:** Internal Medicine
**Program name:** University of Alabama Medical Center (Huntsville) Program
**Program code:** 140-01-00-893
**State:** Alabama
**Address:** University of Alabama School of Med Huntsville, Internal Medicine Program,
          301 Governors Dr SW, Huntsville, AL 35801
**Phone:** (256) 551-4608
**Fax:** (256) 551-4619
**Percentage of IMGs in the program:** 4%
**Minimum USMLE Step 1 Score Requirement:** 210
**Minimum USMLE Step 2 Score Requirement:** 220
**Attempts on any step:** Must pass on first attempt including CS exam
**CS required at time of application:** Yes
**USCE Requirement:** None
**Cut-Off time since graduation:** 5 years
**Program offers couple match:** Yes
**Visas Sponsored or accepted:** J1 visa and H1b visa

## University of Alabama Medical Center (Montgomery) Internal Medicine Residency Program

**Specialty:** Internal Medicine

**Program name:** University of Alabama Medical Center (Montgomery) Program
**Program code:** 140-01-21-447
**NRMP Code:** 1009140C0, 1009140P0
**Program type:** Community-based university affiliated hospital
**State:** Alabama
**Address:** UAB Health Center Montgomery, Internal Medicine Program Suite 200
          2055 E South Blvd, Montgomery, AL 36116-2975
**Phone:** (334) 551-2002
**Fax:** (334) 284-9020
**Percentage of IMGs in the program:** 55%
**Minimum USMLE Step 1 Score Requirement:** 194
**Minimum USMLE Step 2 Score Requirement:** 203
**Attempts on any step:** No limits set
**CS required at time of application:** No
**USCE Requirement:** None
**Cut-Off time since graduation:** No limits set
**Program offers couple match:** No
**Visas Sponsored or accepted:** J1 visa and H1b visa

## University of South Alabama Internal Medicine Residency Program

**Specialty:** Internal Medicine
**Program name:** University of South Alabama Program
**Program code:** 140-01-11-024
**NRMP Code:** 1852140C0, 1852140P0, 1852140P1
**Program type:** University-based
**State:** Alabama
**Address:** University of South Alabama Medical Center, Department of Medicine Mastin 400-L, 2451 Fillingim St, Mobile, AL  36617
**Phone:** (251) 471-7891
**Fax:** (251) 471-1291
**Percentage of IMGs in the program:** 4%
**Minimum USMLE Step 1 Score Requirement:** 219
**Minimum USMLE Step 2 Score Requirement:** 219
**Attempts on any step:** Must pass on first attempt including CS exam
**CS required at time of application:** Yes including ECFMG certificate
**USCE Requirement:** 3 months
**Cut-Off time since graduation:** Recent graduates only
**Program offers couple match:** Yes
**Visas Sponsored or accepted:** J1 visa

# University of Alabama Medical Center Internal Medicine Residency Program

**Specialty:** Internal Medicine
**Program name:** University of Alabama Medical Center Program
**Program code:** 140-01-21-022
**NRMP Code:** 1007140P0, 1007140C2, 1007140C0
**Program type:** University-based
**State:** Alabama
**Address:** University of Alabama Medical Center, BDB 321,
        1720 2nd Ave S, Birmingham, AL 35294-0012
**Phone:** (205) 934-9666
**Fax:** (205) 975-6424
**Percentage of IMGs in the program:** 5%
**Minimum USMLE Step 1 Score Requirement:** 210
**Minimum USMLE Step 2 Score Requirement:** 220
**Attempts on any step:** Must pass first attempt on any step including CS
**CS required at time of application:** No
**USCE Requirement:** None
**Cut-Off time since graduation:** 5 years
**Program offers couple match:** Yes

**Visas Sponsored or accepted:** J1 visa and H1b visa

## Baptist Health System Internal Medicine Residency Program

**Specialty:** Internal Medicine
**Program name:** Baptist Health System Program
**Program code:** 140-01-21-020
**NRMP Code:** 1903140C0, 1903140P0
**Program type:** Community-based
**State:** Alabama
**Address:** Trinity Medical Center, Suite 317,
840 Montclair Rd, Birmingham, AL 35213
**Phone:** (205) 592-5745
**Fax:** (205) 599-4702
**Percentage of IMGs in the program:** 15%
**Minimum USMLE Step 1 Score Requirement:** 205
**Minimum USMLE Step 2 Score Requirement:** 205
**Attempts on any step:** Must pass on first attempt including CS exam
**CS required at time of application:** Yes including ECFMG certificate
**USCE Requirement:** None
**Cut-Off time since graduation:** 3 years
**Program offers couple match:** Yes

**Visas Sponsored or accepted:** J1 visa

## Arizona

## St Joseph's Hospital and Medical Center Internal Medicine Residency Program

**Specialty:** Internal Medicine
**Program name:**St Joseph's Hospital and Medical Center Program
**Program code:** 140-03-11-027
**NRMP Code:** 1012140C0
**Program type:** Community-based university affiliated hospital
**State:** Arizona
**Address:** St Joseph's Hospital and Medical Center, Department of Medicine Suite 900,
        500 W Thomas Rd, Phoenix, AZ  85013
**Phone:** (602) 406-3915
**Fax:** (602) 294-5033
**Percentage of IMGs in the program:** 20%
**Minimum USMLE Step 1 Score Requirement:** 210
**Minimum USMLE Step 2 Score Requirement:** 210

**Attempts on any step:** Must pass on first attempt
**CS required at time of application:** No
**USCE Requirement:** Yes, 6 months
**Cut-Off time since graduation:** 5 years
**Program offers couple match:** Yes
**Visas Sponsored or accepted:** J1 visa

## University of Arizona College of Medicine at South Campus Internal Medicine Residency Program

**Specialty:** Internal Medicine
**Program name:** University of Arizona College of Medicine at South Campus Program
**Program code:** 140-03-12-536
**State:** Arizona
**Address:** University of Arizona College of Medicine-South Campus, Internal Medicine Program,
    2800 E Ajo Way, Tucson, AZ  85713
**Phone:** (520) 874-4502
**Fax:** (520) 874-4510
**Percentage of IMGs in the program:** 90%
**Minimum USMLE Step 1 Score Requirement:** No limits set
**Minimum USMLE Step 2 Score Requirement:** No limits set
**Attempts on any step:** No limits set

**CS required at time of application:** No
**USCE Requirement:** None
**Cut-Off time since graduation:** 5 years
**Program offers couple match:** Yes
**Visas Sponsored or accepted:** J1 visa

## University of Arizona Internal Medicine Residency Program

**Specialty:** Internal Medicine
**Program name:** University of Arizona Program
**Program code:** 140-03-21-029
**NRMP Code:** 1015140P0, 1015140C0
**Program type:** University-based
**State:** Arizona
**Address:** University of Arizona Health Sciences Center, PO Box 245040,
           1501 N Campbell Ave, Tucson, AZ 85724-5040
**Phone:** (520) 626-2761
**Fax:** (520) 626-6020
**Percentage of IMGs in the program:** 40%
**Minimum USMLE Step 1 Score Requirement:** 210
**Minimum USMLE Step 2 Score Requirement:** 210
**Attempts on any step:** No limits set
**CS required at time of application:** No

**USCE Requirement:** Yes 2 months
**Cut-Off time since graduation:** 5 years
**Program offers couple match:** Yes
**Visas Sponsored or accepted:** J1 visa

## Maricopa Medical Center Internal Medicine Residency Program

**Specialty:** Internal Medicine
**Program name:** Maricopa Medical Center Program
**Program code:** 140-03-11-026
**NRMP Code:** 1898140C0, 1898140P0
**Program type:** Community-based university affiliated hospital
**State:** Arizona
**Address:** Maricopa Medical Center, Department of Medicine #OD10,
         2601 E Roosevelt St, Phoenix, AZ 85008
**Phone:** (602) 344-1218
**Fax:** (602) 344-1488
**Percentage of IMGs in the program:** 20%
**Minimum USMLE Step 1 Score Requirement:** 206
**Minimum USMLE Step 2 Score Requirement:** 206

**Attempts on any step:** Must pass on first attempt including CS exam
**CS required at time of application:** Yes
**USCE Requirement:** Yes, 2 months
**Cut-Off time since graduation:** 5 years
**Program offers couple match:** Yes
**Visas Sponsored or accepted:** No visa

## Banner Good Samaritan Medical Center Internal Medicine Residency Program

**Specialty:** Internal Medicine
**Program name:** Banner Good Samaritan Medical Center Program
**Program code:** 140-03-21-025
**NRMP Code:** 1011140C0, 1011140P0
**Program type:** Community-based university affiliated hospital
**State:** Arizona
**Address:** Banner Good Samaritan Medical Center, Department of Internal Medicine,
        1111 E McDowell Rd, Phoenix, AZ 85006
**Phone:** (602) 839-3644
**Fax:** (602) 839-2084
**Percentage of IMGs in the program:** 10%
**Minimum USMLE Step 1 Score Requirement:** 205

**Minimum USMLE Step 2 Score Requirement:** 205
**Attempts on any step:** Must pass on first attempt
**CS required at time of application:** Yes
**USCE Requirement:** Yes, 1 year.
**Cut-Off time since graduation:** 3 years
**Program offers couple match:** Yes
**Visas Sponsored or accepted:** No visa

# Arkansas

## University of Arkansas for Medical Sciences Internal Medicine Residency Program

**Specialty:** Internal Medicine Residency
**Program name:** University of Arkansas for Medical Sciences Program
**Program code:** 140-04-21-030
**NRMP Code:** 1018140C0, 1018140P0
**Program type:** University-based
**State:** Arkansas
**Address:** University of Arkansas for Medical Sciences, Internal Medicine Program Office 634,

4301 W Markham St, Little Rock, AR 72205-7199
**Phone:** (501) 686-5162
**Fax:** (501) 686-6001
**Percentage of IMGs in the program:** 35%
**Minimum USMLE Step 1 Score Requirement:** 210
**Minimum USMLE Step 2 Score Requirement:** 220
**Attempts on any step:** Must pass on first attempt
**CS required at time of application:** Yes including ECFMG cettificate
**USCE Requirement:** None
**Cut-Off time since graduation:** 7 years
**Program offers couple match:** Yes
**Visas Sponsored or accepted:** J1 visa and H1b visa

## California

## University of California Riverside School of Medicine Internal Medicine Residency Program

**Specialty:** Internal Medicine
**Program name:** University of California Riverside School of Medicine Program
**Program code:** 140-05-00-903
**Program type:** University-based
**State:** California
**Address:** Riverside County Regional Medical Center, Internal Medicine Program,
          26250 Cactus Ave, Moreno Valley, CA 92555
**Phone:** (951) 827-7669
**Fax:** (951) 486-4645
**Percentage of IMGs in the program:** 60%
**Minimum USMLE Step 1 Score Requirement:** 200
**Minimum USMLE Step 2 Score Requirement:** 205
**Attempts on any step:** No limits set
**CS required at time of application:** Yes including ECFMG certificate and PTAL/Status letter
**USCE Requirement:** None
**Cut-Off time since graduation:** 5 years
**Program offers couple match:** Yes
**Visas Sponsored or accepted:** J1 visa


Eisenhower Medical Center Internal Medicine Residency Program

**Specialty:** Internal Medicine
**Program name:** Eisenhower Medical Center Program
**Program code:** 140-05-00-895
**Program type:** Community-based University affiliated hospital
**State:** California
**Address:** Eisenhower Medical Center, Internal Medicine Program,
          39000 Bob Hope Dr, Rancho Mirage, CA  92270
**Phone:** (760) 773-2036
**Fax:** (760) 837-8581
**Percentage of IMGs in the program:** 20%
**Minimum USMLE Step 1 Score Requirement:** 210
**Minimum USMLE Step 2 Score Requirement:** 210
**Attempts on any step:** Must pass on first attempt including CS exam
**CS required at time of application:** Yes including ECFMG certificate and PTAL/Status letter
**USCE Requirement:** None
**Cut-Off time since graduation:** 5 years
**Program offers couple match:** Yes
**Visas Sponsored or accepted:** No visa

# Los Angeles County-Harbor-UCLA Medical Center Program

**Specialty:** Internal Medicine
**Program name:** Los Angeles County-Harbor-UCLA Medical Center Program
**Program code:** 140-05-11-070
**State:** California
**Address:** Los Angeles County-Harbor-UCLA Medical Center, Box 400,
            1000 W Carson St, Torrance, CA 90509
**Phone:** (310) 222-2401
**Fax:** (310) 320-9688
**Percentage of IMGs in the program:** 0% (occasional IMG out of the match when a spot is open)
**Minimum USMLE Step 1 Score Requirement:** No limits set
**Minimum USMLE Step 2 Score Requirement:** No limits set
**Attempts on any step:** No limits set
**CS required at time of application:** No but PTAL/Status letter is required
**USCE Requirement:** None
**Cut-Off time since graduation:** No limits set
**Program offers couple match:** Yes
**Visas Sponsored or accepted:** No visa

# Kaiser Permanente Medical Group (Northern California)/Santa Clara Internal Medicine Residency Program

**Specialty:** Internal Medicine
**Program name:** Kaiser Permanente Medical Group (Northern California)/Santa Clara Program
**Program code:** 140-05-21-067
**NRMP Code:** 2135140C1, 2135140P0, 2135140C0
**Program type:** Community-based university affiliated hospital
**State:** California
**Address:** Kaiser Permanente Santa Clara, Graduate Medical Education Department 384, 710 Lawrence Expressway, Santa Clara, CA 95051-5386
**Phone:** (408) 851-3834
**Fax:** (408) 851-3839
**Percentage of IMGs in the program:** 10%
**Minimum USMLE Step 1 Score Requirement:** No limits set
**Minimum USMLE Step 2 Score Requirement:** No limits set
**Attempts on any step:** No limits set

**CS required at time of application:** Yes including ECFMG certificate and PTAL/Status letter
**USCE Requirement:** None
**Cut-Off time since graduation:** 5 years
**Program offers couple match:** Yes
**Visas Sponsored or accepted:** No visa

## Santa Barbara Cottage Hospital Internal Medicine Residency Program

**Specialty:** Internal Medicine
**Program name:** Santa Barbara Cottage Hospital Program
**Program code:** 140-05-22-066
**NRMP Code:** 1064140P0, 1064140C0
**Program type:** Community-based
**State:** California
**Address:** Santa Barbara Cottage Hospital, PO Box 689,
400 W Pueblo St, Santa Barbara, CA 93102
**Phone:** (805) 569-7315
**Fax:** (805) 569-8358
**Percentage of IMGs in the program:** 60%
**Minimum USMLE Step 1 Score Requirement:** No limits set

**Minimum USMLE Step 2 Score Requirement:** No limits set
**Attempts on any step:** Must pass on first attempt including CS exam
**CS required at time of application:** Yes including ECFMG certificate and PTAL/Status letter
**USCE Requirement:** None
**Cut-Off time since graduation:** 3 years unless clinically active
**Program offers couple match:** Yes
**Visas Sponsored or accepted:** J1 visa

## St Mary's Hospital and Medical Center Internal Medicine Residency Program

**Specialty:** Internal Medicine
**Program name:** St Mary's Hospital and Medical Center Program
**Program code:** 140-05-22-063
**NRMP Code:** 1057140C0, 1057140P0
**Program type:** Community-based university affiliated hospital
**State:** California
**Address:** St Mary's Medical Center, Medical Education Department,

450 Stanyan St, San Francisco, CA 94117
**Phone**: (415) 750-5955
**Fax:** (415) 750-8149
**Percentage of IMGs in the program:** 20%
**Minimum USMLE Step 1 Score Requirement:** 220
**Minimum USMLE Step 2 Score Requirement:** 220
**Attempts on any step:** Must pass on first attempt including CS exam
**CS required at time of application:** Yes including ECFMG certificate and PTAL/Status letter
**USCE Requirement:** Yes
**Cut-Off time since graduation:** 3 years
**Program offers couple match:** Yes
**Visas Sponsored or accepted:** No visa

## Huntington Memorial Hospital Internal Medicine Residency Program

**Specialty:** Internal Medicine
**Program name:** Huntington Memorial Hospital Program
**Program code:** 140-05-11-056
**NRMP Code:** 1044140P0, 1044140C0

**Program type:** Community-based university affiliated hospital
**State:** California
**Address:** Huntington Memorial Hospital, Medical Education Department La Vina Bldg, 100 W California Blvd, Pasadena, CA 91109-7013
**Phone:** (626) 397-5188
**Fax:** (626) 397-2914
**Percentage of IMGs in the program:** 3%
**Minimum USMLE Step 1 Score Requirement:** No limits set
**Minimum USMLE Step 2 Score Requirement:** No limits set
**Attempts on any step:** Must pass on first attempt including CS exam
**CS required at time of application:** Yes including ECFMG certificate and PTAL/Status letter
**USCE Requirement:** None
**Cut-Off time since graduation:** 5 years
**Program offers couple match:** Yes
**Visas Sponsored or accepted:** No visa

## University of California (Irvine) Internal Medicine Residency Program

**Specialty:** Internal Medicine

**Program name:** University of California (Irvine) Program
**Program code:** 140-05-21-036
**NRMP Code:** 1043140C0, 1043140P1, 1043140P0
**Program type:** University-based
**State:** California
**Address:** UC Irvine Medical Center, City Tower Suite 400,
　　　101 The City Dr S, Orange, CA  92868
**Phone:** (714) 456-5691
**Fax:** (714) 456-8874
**Percentage of IMGs in the program:** 3%
**Minimum USMLE Step 1 Score Requirement:** 210
**Minimum USMLE Step 2 Score Requirement:** 210
**Attempts on any step:** Must pass on first attempt including CS exam
**CS required at time of application:** Yes including ECFMG certificate and PTAL/Status letter
**USCE Requirement:** None
**Cut-Off time since graduation:** 3 years
**Program offers couple match:** Yes
**Visas Sponsored or accepted:** No visa

# Alameda County Medical Center Internal Medicine Residency Program

**Specialty:** Internal Medicine
**Program name:** Alameda County Medical Center Program
**Program code:** 140-05-31-051
**NRMP Code:** 1041140P0, 1041140M0, 1041140C0
**Program type:** Community-based
**State:** California
**Address:** Alameda County Medical Center, Department of Medicine,
        1411 E 31st St, Oakland, CA  94602
**Phone:** (510) 535-7618
**Fax:** (510) 437-5134
**Percentage of IMGs in the program:** 60%
**Minimum USMLE Step 1 Score Requirement:** No limits set
**Minimum USMLE Step 2 Score Requirement:** No limits set
**Attempts on any step:** No limits set
**CS required at time of application:** Yes including ECFMG certificate and PTAL/Status letter
**USCE Requirement:** None
**Cut-Off time since graduation:** No limits set
**Program offers couple match:** Yes
**Visas Sponsored or accepted:** No visa

# White Memorial Medical Center Internal Medicine Residency Program

**Specialty:** Internal Medicine
**Program name:** White Memorial Medical Center Program
**Program code:** 140-05-11-049
**State:** California
**Address:** White Memorial Medical Center, Department of Internal Medicine,
          1720 Cesar E Chavez Ave, Los Angeles, CA 90033-2481
**Phone:** (323) 268-5000   Ext: 1607
**Fax:** (323) 881-8702
**Percentage of IMGs in the program:** 15%
**Minimum USMLE Step 1 Score Requirement:** No limits set
**Minimum USMLE Step 2 Score Requirement:** No limits set
**Attempts on any step:** No limits set
**CS required at time of application:** Yes including ECFMG certificate and PTAL/Status letter
**USCE Requirement:** None
**Cut-Off time since graduation:** 7 years
**Program offers couple match:** Yes

**Visas Sponsored or accepted:** J1 visa

## Kaiser Permanente Southern California (Los Angeles) Internal Medicine Residency Program

**Specialty:** Internal Medicine
**Program name:** Kaiser Permanente Southern California (Los Angeles) Program
**Program code:** 140-05-12-042
**State:** California
**Address:** Kaiser Permanente Medical Care, Residency Admin & Recruitment 5th Fl,
            393 E Walnut St, Pasadena, CA  91188
**Phone:** (877) 574-0002
**Fax:** (626) 405-6581
**Percentage of IMGs in the program:** 8%
**Minimum USMLE Step 1 Score Requirement:** No limits set
**Minimum USMLE Step 2 Score Requirement:** No limits set
**Attempts on any step:** Must pass on first attempt
**CS required at time of application:** Yes including ECFMG certificate and PTAL/Status letter
**USCE Requirement:** None
**Cut-Off time since graduation:** No limits set
**Program offers couple match:** Yes

**Visas Sponsored or accepted:** No visa

## St Mary Medical Center Internal Medicine Residency Program

**Specialty:** Internal Medicine
**Program name:** St Mary Medical Center Program
**Program code:** 140-05-31-039
**State:** California
**Address:** St Mary Medical Center, Department of Internal Medicine,
          1050 Linden Ave, Long Beach, CA 90813
**Phone:** (562) 491-9000    Ext:  2356
**Fax:**  (562) 491-9146
**Percentage of IMGs in the program:** 25%
**Minimum USMLE Step 1 Score Requirement:** 200
**Minimum USMLE Step 2 Score Requirement:** 205
**Attempts on any step:** No limits set
**CS required at time of application:** Yes including ECFMG certificate and PTAL/Status letter
**USCE Requirement:** Yes
**Cut-Off time since graduation:** 4 years
**Program offers couple match:** Yes
**Visas Sponsored or accepted:** J1 visa

## Loma Linda University Internal Medicine Residency Program

**Specialty:** Internal Medicine
**Program name:** Loma Linda University Program
**Program code:** 140-05-21-038
**NRMP Code:** 1024140C0, 1024140P0, 1024140M0
**Program type:** University-based
**State:** California
**Address:** Loma Linda University Medical Center, Rm 1503,
        11234 Anderson St, Loma Linda, CA 92354
**Phone:** (909) 558-4074
**Fax:** (909) 558-0427
**Percentage of IMGs in the program:** 20%
**Minimum USMLE Step 1 Score Requirement:** No limits set
**Minimum USMLE Step 2 Score Requirement:** No limits set
**Attempts on any step:** Must pass on first attempt
**CS required at time of application:** Yes including ECFMG certificate and PTAL/Status letter
**USCE Requirement:** None
**Cut-Off time since graduation:** 7 years unless clinically active
**Program offers couple match:** Yes

**Visas Sponsored or accepted:** ECFMG J1 visa or H1b visa from medical school for AMGs

## Scripps Clinic/Scripps Green Hospital Internal Medicine Residency Program

**Specialty:** Internal Medicine
**Program name:** Scripps Clinic/Scripps Green Hospital Program
**Program code:** 140-05-21-490
**NRMP Code:** 1340140C0, 1340140C1
**Program type:** Community-based university affiliated hospital
**State:** California
**Address:** Scripps Clinic/Scripps Green Hospital, Department of Graduate Medical Education Suite 403C,
10666 N Torrey Pines Rd, La Jolla, CA 92037-1093
**Phone:** (858) 554-3200
**Percentage of IMGs in the program:** 8%
**Minimum USMLE Step 1 Score Requirement:** 200
**Minimum USMLE Step 2 Score Requirement:** 220
**Attempts on any step:** Must pass on first attempt including CS exam

**CS required at time of application:** Yes including ECFMG certificate and PTAL/Status letter
**USCE Requirement:** Yes
**Cut-Off time since graduation:** 10 years
**Program offers couple match:** Yes
**Visas Sponsored or accepted:** No visa

## University of California (San Francisco)/Fresno Internal Medicine Residency Program

**Specialty:** Internal Medicine
**Program name:** University of California (San Francisco)/Fresno Program
**Program code:** 140-05-31-033
**State:** California
**Address:** UCSF Fresno, Internal Medicine Program Suite 301,
155 N Fresno St, Fresno, CA  93701
**Phone:** (559) 499-6479
**Fax:** (559) 499-6501
**Percentage of IMGs in the program:** 30%
**Minimum USMLE Step 1 Score Requirement:** No limits set
**Minimum USMLE Step 2 Score Requirement:** No limits set
**Attempts on any step:** Must pass on first attempt including CS exam

**CS required at time of application:** Yes including PTAL/Status letter.
**USCE Requirement:** None
**Cut-Off time since graduation:** 5 years
**Program offers couple match:** Yes
**Visas Sponsored or accepted:** J1 visa

## San Joaquin General Hospital Internal Medicine Residency Program

**Specialty:** Internal Medicine
**Program name:** San Joaquin General Hospital Program
**Program code:** 140-05-12-069
**State:** California
**Address:** San Joaquin General Hospital, Internal Medicine Pgm GME Office,
          500 W Hospital Rd, French Camp, CA 95231
**Phone:** (209) 468-6624
**Fax:** (209) 468-6246
**Percentage of IMGs in the program:** 85%
**Minimum USMLE Step 1 Score Requirement:** 205
**Minimum USMLE Step 2 Score Requirement:** 205

**Attempts on any step:** Must pass on first attempt
**CS required at time of application:** No but PTAL/Status letter is required
**USCE Requirement:** None
**Cut-Off time since graduation:** 3 years
**Program offers couple match:** Yes
**Visas Sponsored or accepted:** J1 visa

## Kern Medical Center Internal Medicine Residency Program

**Specialty:** Internal Medicine
**Program name:** Kern Medical Center Program
**Program code:** 140-05-31-031
**NRMP Code:** 1921140C0
**Program type:** Community-based university affiliated hospital
**State:** California
**Address:** Kern Medical Center, Department of Medicine,
          1700 Mount Vernon Ave, Bakersfield, CA  93306
**Phone:** (661) 326-2202
**Fax:** (661) 862-7612
**Percentage of IMGs in the program:** 100%
**Minimum USMLE Step 1 Score Requirement:** 200

**Minimum USMLE Step 2 Score Requirement:** 205
**Attempts on any step:** Must pass on first attempt
**CS required at time of application:** Yes including ECFMG certificate and PTAL/Status letter
**USCE Requirement:** None
**Cut-Off time since graduation:** 5 years
**Program offers couple match:** Yes
**Visas Sponsored or accepted:** J1 visa and H1b visa

# Colorado

## Exempla St Joseph Hospital Internal Medicine Residency Program

**Specialty:** Internal Medicine
**Program name:** Exempla St Joseph Hospital Program
**Program code:** 140-07-31-072
**State:** Colorado
**Address:** Exempla St Joseph Hospital,
      1835 Franklin St, Denver, CO 80218
**Phone:** (303) 837-7837

**Fax:** (303) 866-8044
**Percentage of IMGs in the program:** 12%
**Minimum USMLE Step 1 Score Requirement:** 205
**Minimum USMLE Step 2 Score Requirement:** 205
**Attempts on any step:** Must pass on first attempt including CS exam
**CS required at time of application:** No
**USCE Requirement:** Yes 2 months
**Cut-Off time since graduation:** 4 years
**Program offers couple match:** Yes
**Visas Sponsored or accepted:** J1 visa and H1b visa

## Connecticut

### Norwalk Hospital/Yale University Internal Medicine Residency Program

**Specialty:** Internal Medicine
**Program name:** Norwalk Hospital/Yale University Program
**Program code:** 140-08-31-086
**NRMP Code:** 1093140C0, 1093140P0
**Program type:** Community-based university

affiliated hospital
**State:** Connecticut
**Address:** Norwalk Hospital,
          34 Maple St, Norwalk, CT  06856
**Phone:** (203) 852-2025
**Fax:** (203) 855-3589
**Percentage of IMGs in the program:** 30%
**Minimum USMLE Step 1 Score Requirement:** 210
**Minimum USMLE Step 2 Score Requirement:** 210
**Attempts on any step:** No limits set
**CS required at time of application:** No
**USCE Requirement:** None
**Cut-Off time since graduation:** No limits set
**Program offers couple match:** Yes
**Visas Sponsored or accepted:** J1 visa and H1b visa

## Yale-New Haven Medical Center (St Raphael) Internal Medicine Residency Program

**Specialty:** Internal Medicine
**Program name:** Yale-New Haven Medical Center (St Raphael) Program
**Program code:** 140-08-31-084
**NRMP Code:** 1090140C0, 1090140P0
**Program type:** Community-based University

affiliated hospital
**State:** Connecticut
**Address:** Hospital of St Raphael
          1450 Chapel St, New Haven, CT  06511
**Phone:** (203) 789-3358
**Fax:** (203) 789-3222
**Percentage of IMGs in the program:** 40%
**Minimum USMLE Step 1 Score Requirement:** 205
**Minimum USMLE Step 2 Score Requirement:** 205
**Attempts on any step:** Must pass on first attempt including CS exam
**CS required at time of application:** Yes including ECFMG certificate
**USCE Requirement:** Yes 2 months
**Cut-Off time since graduation:** 6 years
**Program offers couple match:** Yes
**Visas Sponsored or accepted:** J1 visa and H1b visa

## University of Connecticut Internal Medicine Residency Program

**Specialty:** Internal Medicine
**Program name:** University of Connecticut Program
**Program code:** 140-08-31-078

**NRMP Code:** 1094140C0, 1094140P0
**Program type:** University-based
**State:** Connecticut
**Address:** University of Connecticut Health
Center

      263 Farmington Ave, Farmington, CT
06030-1235
**Phone:** (860) 679-2562
**Fax:** (860) 679-4613
**Percentage of IMGs in the program:** 50%
**Minimum USMLE Step 1 Score Requirement:**
205
**Minimum USMLE Step 2 Score Requirement:**
205
**Attempts on any step:** No limits set
**CS required at time of application:** No
**USCE Requirement:** None
**Cut-Off time since graduation:** 5 years
**Program offers couple match:** Yes
**Visas Sponsored or accepted:** J1 visa


## Griffin Hospital Internal Medicine Residency Program

**Specialty:** Internal Medicine
**Program name:** Griffin Hospital Program
**Program code:** 140-08-31-077
**NRMP Code:** 1977140P0, 1977140C0
**Program type:** Community-based university

affiliated hospital
**State:** Connecticut
**Address:** Griffin Hospital
          130 Division St, Derby, CT  06418
**Phone:** (203) 732-7327
**Fax:** (203) 732-7185
**Percentage of IMGs in the program:** 80%
**Minimum USMLE Step 1 Score Requirement:** 220
**Minimum USMLE Step 2 Score Requirement:** 220
**Attempts on any step:** Pass on 2nd attempt max.
**CS required at time of application:** Yes
**USCE Requirement:** None
**Cut-Off time since graduation:** 5 years
**Program offers couple match:** No
**Visas Sponsored or accepted:** J1 visa and H1b visa

## University of Connecticut (New Britain) Internal Medicine Residency Program

**Specialty:** Internal Medicine
**Program name:** University of Connecticut (New Britain) Program
**Program code:** 140-08-21-499

**NRMP Code:** 1094140M0
**Program type:** University-based
**State:** Connecticut
**Address:** University of Connecticut Health Center
          263 Farmington Ave, Farmington, CT 06030-1234
**Phone:** (860) 679-4017
**Fax:** (860) 679-1621
**Percentage of IMGs in the program:** 60%
**Minimum USMLE Step 1 Score Requirement:** 205
**Minimum USMLE Step 2 Score Requirement:** 205
**Attempts on any step:** Must pass on first attempt including CS exam
**CS required at time of application:** No
**USCE Requirement:** None
**Cut-Off time since graduation:** 5 years
**Program offers couple match:** Yes
**Visas Sponsored or accepted:** J1 visa

## Yale-New Haven Medical Center Internal Medicine Residency Program

**Specialty:** Internal Medicine
**Program name:** Yale-New Haven Medical Center Program
**Program code:** 140-08-21-085

**NRMP Code:** 1089140C1, 1089140P0, 1089140P2, 1089140C0
**Program type:** University-based
**State:** Connecticut
**Address:** Yale-New Haven Medical Center
15 York St, New Haven, CT  06520-8030
**Phone:** (203) 785-4123
**Percentage of IMGs in the program:** 5%
**Minimum USMLE Step 1 Score Requirement:** 230
**Minimum USMLE Step 2 Score Requirement:** 230
**Attempts on any step:** Must pass on first attempt including CS exam
**CS required at time of application:** Yes
**USCE Requirement:** Yes 2 months
**Cut-Off time since graduation:** 6 years
**Program offers couple match:** Yes
**Visas Sponsored or accepted:** J1 visa and H1b visa

## Yale-New Haven Hospital Internal Medicine Residency Program

**Specialty:** Internal Medicine
**Program name:** Yale-New Haven Hospital Program

**Program code:** 140-08-00-910
**Program type:** University-based
**State:** Connecticut
**Address:** Waterburg Hospital
         64 Robbins St, Waterbury, CT 06708
**Phone:** (203) 573-6574
**Fax:** (203) 573-6707
**Percentage of IMGs in the program:** 10%
**Minimum USMLE Step 1 Score Requirement:** 220
**Minimum USMLE Step 2 Score Requirement:** 220
**Attempts on any step:** Must pass on first attempt
**CS required at time of application:** Yes
**USCE Requirement:** Yes 2 months
**Cut-Off time since graduation:** 5 years
**Program offers couple match:** Yes
**Visas Sponsored or accepted:** J1 visa and H1b visa

## St. Vincent Medical Center Internal Medicine Residency Program

**Specialty:** Internal Medicine
**Program name:** St. Vincent Medical Center Program
**Program code:** 140-08-11-075
**NRMP Code:** 1080140P0, 1080140C0
**Program type:** Community-based university

affiliated hospital
**State:** Connecticut
**Address:** St Vincent's Medical Center
          2800 Main St, Bridgeport, CT  06606
**Phone:** (203) 576-5576
**Percentage of IMGs in the program:** 85%
**Minimum USMLE Step 1 Score Requirement:** 210
**Minimum USMLE Step 2 Score Requirement:** 210
**Attempts on any step:** No limits set
**CS required at time of application:** Yes
**USCE Requirement:** Yes 2 months
**Cut-Off time since graduation:** 10 years
**Program offers couple match:** Yes
**Visas Sponsored or accepted:** J1 visa and H1b visa

## Greenwich Hospital Association Internal Medicine Residency Program

**Specialty:** Internal Medicine
**Program name:** Greenwich Hospital Association Program
**Program code:** 140-08-21-079
**NRMP Code:** 1082140C0, 1082140P0
**Program type:** Community-based university affiliated hospital
**State:** Connecticut

**Address:** Greenwich Hospital
        5 Perryridge Rd, Greenwich, CT  06830
**Phone:** (203) 863-3913
**Fax:** (203) 863-3924
**Percentage of IMGs in the program:** 20%
**Minimum USMLE Step 1 Score Requirement:**
230
**Minimum USMLE Step 2 Score Requirement:**
230
**Attempts on any step:** Must pass on first
attempt
**CS required at time of application:** No
**USCE Requirement:** None
**Cut-Off time since graduation:** 5 years
**Program offers couple match:** Yes
**Visas Sponsored or accepted:** J1 visa and H1b
visa

## St. Mary Hospital (Waterbury) Internal Medicine Residency Program

**Specialty:** Internal Medicine
**Program name:** St. Mary Hospital (Waterbury)
Program
**Program code:** 140-08-13-530
**NRMP Code:** 1096140P0, 1096140C0
**Program type:** Community-based University
affiliated hospital
**State:** Connecticut

**Address:** St Mary's Hospital
        56 Franklin St, Waterbury, CT  06706
**Phone:** (203) 709-6424
**Fax:** (203) 709-3518
**Percentage of IMGs in the program:** 85%
**Minimum USMLE Step 1 Score Requirement:** 206
**Minimum USMLE Step 2 Score Requirement:** 206
**Attempts on any step:** Must pass on first attempt
**CS required at time of application:** No
**USCE Requirement:** Yes 1 month
**Cut-Off time since graduation:** 3 years
**Program offers couple match:** Yes
**Visas Sponsored or accepted:** J1 visa


## Stamford Hospital/Columbia University College of Physicians and Surgeons Internal Medicine Residency Program

**Specialty:** Internal Medicine
**Program name:** Stamford Hospital/Columbia University College of Physicians and Surgeons Program
**Program code:** 140-08-11-087
**NRMP Code:** 1095140C0, 1095140P0
**Program type:** Community-based university

affiliated hospital
**State:** Connecticut
**Address:** Stamford Hospital
        30 Shelburne Rd, Stamford, CT  06904
**Phone:** (203) 276-7147
**Fax:** (203) 276-7368
**Percentage of IMGs in the program:** 35%
**Minimum USMLE Step 1 Score Requirement:** 210
**Minimum USMLE Step 2 Score Requirement:** 210
**Attempts on any step:** Must pass on first attempt
**CS required at time of application:** Yes
**USCE Requirement:** Yes
**Cut-Off time since graduation:** No limits set
**Program offers couple match:** Yes
**Visas Sponsored or accepted:** No visa

## Danbury Hospital Internal Medicine Residency Program

**Specialty:** Internal Medicine
**Program name:** Danbury Hospital Program
**Program code:** 140-08-11-076
**NRMP Code:** 1081140C1, 1081140C0
**Program type:** Community-based university affiliated hospital
**State:** Connecticut

**Address:** Danbury Hospital
            24 Hospital Ave, Danbury, CT  06810
**Phone:** (203) 739-8048
**Fax:** (203) 739-4912
**Percentage of IMGs in the program:** 85%
**Minimum USMLE Step 1 Score Requirement:** 210
**Minimum USMLE Step 2 Score Requirement:** 210
**Attempts on any step:** No limits set
**CS required at time of application:** No
**USCE Requirement:** None
**Cut-Off time since graduation:** 10 years
**Program offers couple match:** Yes
**Visas Sponsored or accepted:** J1 visa and H1b visa

## Bridgeport Hospital/Yale University Internal Medicine Residency Program

**Specialty:** Internal Medicine
**Program name:** Bridgeport Hospital/Yale University Program
**Program code:** 140-08-11-074
**NRMP Code:** 1079140C0
**Program type:** Community-based university affiliated hospital
**State:** Connecticut

**Address:** Bridgeport Hospital
            267 Grant St, Bridgeport, CT  06610
**Phone:** (203) 384-3792
**Fax:** (203) 384-4294
**Percentage of IMGs in the program:** 80%
**Minimum USMLE Step 1 Score Requirement:** 210
**Minimum USMLE Step 2 Score Requirement:** 210
**Attempts on any step:** Must pass on first attempt including CS exam
**CS required at time of application:** Yes
**USCE Requirement:** Yes 3 months
**Cut-Off time since graduation:** 5 years
**Program offers couple match:** Yes
**Visas Sponsored or accepted:** J1 visa and H1b visa

# Delaware

## Jefferson Medical College/Christiana Care Health Services Internal Medicine Residency Program

**Specialty:** Internal Medicine

**Program name:** Jefferson Medical College/Christiana Care Health Services Program
**Program code:** 140-09-11-090
**NRMP Code:** 1099140C0, 1099140P0
**Program type:** Community-based university affiliated hospital
**State:** Delaware
**Address:** Christiana Care Health System
4755 Ogletown-Stanton Rd, Newark, DE  19718
**Phone:** (302) 733-6338
**Fax:** (302) 733-6386
**Percentage of IMGs in the program:** 15%
**Minimum USMLE Step 1 Score Requirement:** No limits set
**Minimum USMLE Step 2 Score Requirement:** No limits set
**Attempts on any step:** No limits set
**CS required at time of application:** No
**USCE Requirement:** None
**Cut-Off time since graduation:** No limits set
**Program offers couple match:** Yes
**Visas Sponsored or accepted:** J1 visa

# District of Columbia

## Providence Hospital Internal Medicine Residency Program

**Specialty:** Internal Medicine
**Program name:** Providence Hospital Program
**Program code:** 140-10-21-095
**NRMP Code:** 1803140C0
**Program type:** Community-based
**State:** District of Columbia
**Address:** Providence Hospital, Department of Medicine
          1150 Varnum St NE, Washington, DC 20017-2180
**Phone:** (202) 269-7747
**Fax:** (202) 269-7892
**Percentage of IMGs in the program:** 70%
**Minimum USMLE Step 1 Score Requirement:** 230
**Minimum USMLE Step 2 Score Requirement:** 230
**Attempts on any step:** Must pass on first attempt
**CS required at time of application:** Yes
**USCE Requirement:** None
**Cut-Off time since graduation:** 5 years unless clinically active can be more
**Program offers couple match:** No
**Visas Sponsored or accepted:** J1 visa and H1b visa

# Howard University Internal Medicine Residency Program

**Specialty:** Internal Medicine
**Program name:** Howard University Program
**Program code:** 140-10-21-461
**Program type:** University-based
**State:** District of Columbia
**Address:** Howard University Hospital, Department of Medicine
          2041 Georgia Ave NW, Washington, DC  20060
**Phone:** (202) 865-1920
**Fax:** (202) 865-7199
**Percentage of IMGs in the program:** 50%
**Minimum USMLE Step 1 Score Requirement:** No limits set
**Minimum USMLE Step 2 Score Requirement:** No limits set
**Attempts on any step:** Maximum of 2 attempts allowed on each step including CS exam
**CS required at time of application:** Yes including ECFMG certificate
**USCE Requirement:** None
**Cut-Off time since graduation:** No limits set
**Program offers couple match:** Yes
**Visas Sponsored or accepted:** J1 visa

# Georgetown University Hospital/Washington Hospital Center Internal Medicine Residency Program

**Specialty:** Internal Medicine
**Program name:** Georgetown University Hospital/Washington Hospital Center Program
**Program code:** 140-10-11-097
**NRMP Code:** 1800140P0, 1800140C0
**Program type:** Community-based university affiliated hospital
**State:** District of Columbia
**Address:** MedStar Washington Hospital Center, Department of Medicine 2A38I
              110 Irving St NW, Washington, DC 20010-2975
**Phone:** (202) 877-8271
**Fax:** (202) 877-6292
**Percentage of IMGs in the program:** 40%
**Minimum USMLE Step 1 Score Requirement:** No limits set
**Minimum USMLE Step 2 Score Requirement:** No limits set
**Attempts on any step:** Must pass on first attempt
**CS required at time of application:** No
**USCE Requirement:** None
**Cut-Off time since graduation:** 5 years
**Program offers couple match:** Yes

**Visas Sponsored or accepted:** J1 visa

# George Washington University Internal Medicine Residency Program

**Specialty:** Internal Medicine
**Program name:** George Washington University Program
**Program code:** 140-10-21-093
**Program type:** University-based
**State:** District of Columbia
**Address:** George Washington University Medical Center, Suite 8-404
2150 Pennsylvania Ave NW, Washington, DC  20037
**Phone:** (202) 741-2235
**Fax:** (202) 741-2241
**Percentage of IMGs in the program:** 20%
**Minimum USMLE Step 1 Score Requirement:** No limits set
**Minimum USMLE Step 2 Score Requirement:** No limits set
**Attempts on any step:** No limits set
**CS required at time of application:** Yes including ECFMG certificate
**USCE Requirement:** Yes 1 month
**Cut-Off time since graduation:** 3 years

**Program offers couple match:** Yes
**Visas Sponsored or accepted:** J1 visa

# Florida

## Florida Hospital Medical Center Internal Medicine Residency Program

**Specialty:** Internal Medicine
**Program name:** Florida Hospital Medical Center Program
**Program code:** 140-11-31-539
**NRMP Code:** 1102140C0
**Program type:** Community-based university affiliated hospital
**State:** Florida
**Address:** Florida Hospital Medical Center
2501 N Orange Ave, Orlando, FL 32804
**Phone:** (407) 303-7331
**Fax:** (407) 303-7285
**Percentage of IMGs in the program:** 50%
**Minimum USMLE Step 1 Score Requirement:**
No limits set
**Minimum USMLE Step 2 Score Requirement:**
No limits set

**Attempts on any step:** Must pass on first attempt
**CS required at time of application:** No
**USCE Requirement:** None
**Cut-Off time since graduation:** No limits set
**Program offers couple match:** Yes
**Visas Sponsored or accepted:** J1 visa and H1b visa

## University of Miami Miller School of Medicine/Palm Beach Regional Campus Internal Medicine Residency Program

**Specialty:** Internal Medicine
**Program name:** University of Miami Miller School of Medicine/Palm Beach Regional Campus Program
**Program code:** 140-11-31-535
**NRMP Code:** 1384140P0, 1384140C0
**Program type:** Community-based university affiliated hospital
**State:** Florida
**Address:** JFK Medical Center
        5301 S Congress Ave, Atlantis, FL 33462
**Phone:** (561) 548-1467
**Fax:** (561) 548-1757
**Percentage of IMGs in the program:** 60%

**Minimum USMLE Step 1 Score Requirement:** 205
**Minimum USMLE Step 2 Score Requirement:** 205
**Attempts on any step:** No limits set
**CS required at time of application:** Yes
**USCE Requirement:** Yes 2 months
**Cut-Off time since graduation:** 5 years
**Program offers couple match:** Yes
**Visas Sponsored or accepted:** J1 visa and H1b visa

## Cleveland Clinic (Florida) Internal Medicine Residency Program

**Specialty:** Internal Medicine
**Program name:** Cleveland Clinic (Florida) Program
**Program code:** 140-11-21-528
**NRMP Code:** 1383140C0, 1383140P0, 1383140P1
**Program type:** Community-based
**State:** Florida
**Address:** Cleveland Clinic Florida
        2950 Cleveland Clinic Blvd, Weston, FL 33331
**Phone:** (954) 659-5884
**Fax:** (954) 659-5622
**Percentage of IMGs in the program:** 70%

**Minimum USMLE Step 1 Score Requirement:** 205

**Minimum USMLE Step 2 Score Requirement:** 205

**Attempts on any step:** Must pass on first attempt including CS exam

**CS required at time of application:** No

**USCE Requirement:** Yes 2 months

**Cut-Off time since graduation:** 3 years

**Program offers couple match:** Yes

**Visas Sponsored or accepted:** J1 visa and H1b visa

## University of South Florida Morsani Internal Medicine Residency Program

**Specialty:** Internal Medicine

**Program name:** University of South Florida Morsani Program

**Program code:** 140-11-21-104

**NRMP Code:** 1109140C0, 1109140P0

**Program type:** University-based

**State:** Florida

**Address:** University of South Florida
17 Davis Blvd, Tampa, FL  33606

**Phone:** (813) 259-0875

**Fax:** (813) 259-0697

**Percentage of IMGs in the program:** 15%

**Minimum USMLE Step 1 Score Requirement:**
220
**Minimum USMLE Step 2 Score Requirement:**
220
**Attempts on any step:** Must pass on first attempt
**CS required at time of application:** Yes including ECFMG certificate
**USCE Requirement:** Yes
**Cut-Off time since graduation:** 3 years
**Program offers couple match:** Yes
**Visas Sponsored or accepted:** J1 visa


## Jackson Memorial Hospital/Jackson Health System Internal Medicine Residency Program

**Specialty:** Internal Medicine
**Program name:** Jackson Memorial Hospital/Jackson Health System Program
**Program code:** 140-11-21-100
**NRMP Code:** 1104140P0, 1104140C0
**Program type:** Community-based University affiliated hospital
**State:** Florida
**Address:** University of Miami Jackson Memorial Hospital
        1611 NW 12th Ave, Miami, FL  33136
**Phone:** (305) 585-5215

**Fax:** (305) 585-8137
**Percentage of IMGs in the program:** 65%
**Minimum USMLE Step 1 Score Requirement:**
No limits set
**Minimum USMLE Step 2 Score Requirement:**
No limits set
**Attempts on any step:** No limits set
**CS required at time of application:** No
**USCE Requirement:** Yes
**Cut-Off time since graduation:** 5 years
**Program offers couple match:** Yes
**Visas Sponsored or accepted:** J1 visa

## University of Florida College of Medicine Jacksonville Internal Medicine Residency Program

**Specialty:** Internal Medicine
**Program name:** University of Florida College of Medicine Jacksonville Program
**Program code:** 140-11-21-099
**NRMP Code:** 1101140P0, 1101140C0
**Program type:** Community-based university affiliated hospital
**State:** Florida
**Address:** University of Florida College of Medicine Jacksonville
          653-1 W 8th St, Jacksonville, FL 32209-6511
**Phone:** (904) 244-3094

**Fax:** (904) 244-4685
**Percentage of IMGs in the program:** 60%
**Minimum USMLE Step 1 Score Requirement:**
No limits set
**Minimum USMLE Step 2 Score Requirement:**
No limits set
**Attempts on any step:** No limits set
**CS required at time of application:** No
**USCE Requirement:** None
**Cut-Off time since graduation:** No limits set
**Program offers couple match:** Yes
**Visas Sponsored or accepted:** J1 visa

## University of Florida Internal Medicine Residency Program

**Specialty:** Internal Medicine
**Program name:** University of Florida Program
**Program code:** 140-11-21-098
**NRMP Code:** 1824140P1, 1824140P0, 1824140C0
**Program type:** University-based
**State:** Florida
**Address:** University of Florida College of Medicine
            1600 SW Archer Rd, Gainesville, FL 32610-0277
**Phone:** (352) 265-0239
**Fax:** (352) 265-1107
**Percentage of IMGs in the program:** 30%

**Minimum USMLE Step 1 Score Requirement:** 220
**Minimum USMLE Step 2 Score Requirement:** 220
**Attempts on any step:** Must pass on first attempt
**CS required at time of application:** No
**USCE Requirement:** Yes
**Cut-Off time since graduation:** 5 years
**Program offers couple match:** Yes
**Visas Sponsored or accepted:** J1 visa

## Mount Sinai Medical Center of Florida Internal Medicine Residency Program

**Specialty:** Internal Medicine
**Program name:** Mount Sinai Medical Center of Florida Program
**Program code:** 140-11-12-101
**NRMP Code:** 1105140P0, 1105140C0
**Program type:** Community-based university affiliated hospital
**State:** Florida
**Address:** Mount Sinai Medical Center Florida
4300 Alton Rd, Miami Beach, FL  33140
**Phone:** (305) 674-2053
**Fax:** (305) 674-2057
**Percentage of IMGs in the program:** 75%

**Minimum USMLE Step 1 Score Requirement:** 210
**Minimum USMLE Step 2 Score Requirement:** 210
**Attempts on any step:** Must pass on first attempt
**CS required at time of application:** No
**USCE Requirement:** None
**Cut-Off time since graduation:** 5 years
**Program offers couple match:** Yes
**Visas Sponsored or accepted:** J1 visa and H1b visa

## Oak Hill Hospital Internal Medicine Residency Program

**Specialty:** Internal Medicine
**Program name:** Oak Hill Hospital Program
**Program code:** 140-11-00-928
**State:** Florida
**Address:** Oak Hill Hospital
        11375 Cortez Blvd, Brooksville, FL 34613
**Phone:** (352) 597-6137
**Fax:** (352) 597-6173
**Percentage of IMGs in the program:** 30%
**Minimum USMLE Step 1 Score Requirement:** No limits set
**Minimum USMLE Step 2 Score Requirement:** No limits set

**Attempts on any step:** Must pass on first attempt
**CS required at time of application:** Yes including ECFMG certificate
**USCE Requirement:** None
**Cut-Off time since graduation:** 2 years
**Program offers couple match:** Yes
**Visas Sponsored or accepted:** No visa

## Aventura Hospital and Medical Center Internal Medicine Residency Program

**Specialty:** Internal Medicine
**Program name:** Aventura Hospital and Medical Center Program
**Program code:** 140-11-00-924
**State:** Florida
**Address:** Aventura Hospital and Medical Center 20900 Biscayne Blvd, Aventura, FL 33180
**Phone:** (305) 682-5293
**Fax:** (305) 682-7105
**Percentage of IMGs in the program:** 50%
**Minimum USMLE Step 1 Score Requirement:** No limits set
**Minimum USMLE Step 2 Score Requirement:** No limits set
**Attempts on any step:** No limits set
**CS required at time of application:** No

**USCE Requirement:** None
**Cut-Off time since graduation:** No limits set
**Program offers couple match:** Yes
**Visas Sponsored or accepted:** J1 visa

## Florida Atlantic University Charles E Schmidt College of Medicine Internal Medicine Residency Program

**Specialty:** Internal Medicine
**Program name:** Florida Atlantic University Charles E Schmidt College of Medicine Program
**Program code:** 140-11-00-923
**Program type:** University-based
**State:** Florida
**Address:** FAU Charles E Schmidt Coll of Med
777 Glades Rd, Boca Raton, FL 33431
**Phone:** (561) 297-0128
**Fax:** (561) 297-2519
**Percentage of IMGs in the program:** 25%
**Minimum USMLE Step 1 Score Requirement:** No limits set
**Minimum USMLE Step 2 Score Requirement:** No limits set
**Attempts on any step:** No limits set
**CS required at time of application:** No
**USCE Requirement:** None
**Cut-Off time since graduation:** No limits set
**Program offers couple match:** Yes

**Visas Sponsored or accepted:** J1 visa

## University of Central Florida College of Medicine Internal Medicine Residency Program

**Specialty:** Internal Medicine
**Program name:** University of Central Florida College of Medicine Program
**Program code:** 140-11-00-909
**Program type:** University-based
**State:** Florida
**Address:** University of Central Florida College of Medicine
        6850 Lake Nona Blvd, Orlando, FL 32827
**Phone:** (407) 266-1106
**Percentage of IMGs in the program:** 40%
**Minimum USMLE Step 1 Score Requirement:** No limits set
**Minimum USMLE Step 2 Score Requirement:** No limits set
**Attempts on any step:** No limits set
**CS required at time of application:** No
**USCE Requirement:** None
**Cut-Off time since graduation:** 5 years
**Program offers couple match:** Yes
**Visas Sponsored or accepted:** J1 visa

# Florida State University College of Medicine Internal Medicine Program

**Specialty:** Internal Medicine
**Program name:** Florida State University College of Medicine Program
**Program code:** 140-11-00-894
**State:** Florida
**Address:** Florida State University College of Medicine

1300 Miccosukee Rd, Tallahassee, FL 32308
**Phone:** (850) 431-7910
**Fax:** (850) 431-8251
**Percentage of IMGs in the program:** 15%
**Minimum USMLE Step 1 Score Requirement:** No limits set
**Minimum USMLE Step 2 Score Requirement:** No limits set
**Attempts on any step:** Must pass on first attempt
**CS required at time of application:** Yes including ECFMG certificate
**USCE Requirement:** None
**Cut-Off time since graduation:** 5 years
**Program offers couple match:** Yes
**Visas Sponsored or accepted:** J1 visa

# Georgia

## Medical Center of Central Georgia/Mercer University School of Medicine Internal Medicine Residency Program

**Specialty:** Internal Medicine
**Program name:** Medical Center of Central Georgia/Mercer University School of Medicine Program
**Program code:** 140-12-21-491
**NRMP Code:** 1120140P0, 1120140C0
**Program type:** Community-based University affiliated hospital
**State:** Georgia
**Address:** Mercer University School of Medicine/MCCG
        707 Pine St, Macon, GA  31201
**Phone:** (478) 301-5824
**Fax:** (478) 301-5825
**Percentage of IMGs in the program:** 50%
**Minimum USMLE Step 1 Score Requirement:** No limits set
**Minimum USMLE Step 2 Score Requirement:** No limits set

**Attempts on any step:** Must pass on first attempt
**CS required at time of application:** No
**USCE Requirement:** Yes
**Cut-Off time since graduation:** 5 years
**Program offers couple match:** Yes
**Visas Sponsored or accepted:** No visa


## Medical College of Georgia Internal Medicine Residency Program

**Specialty:** Internal Medicine
**Program name:** Medical College of Georgia Program
**Program code:** 140-12-21-107
**NRMP Code:** 1985140C0, 1985140P0, 1985140C1
**Program type:** University-based
**State:** Georgia
**Address:** Medical College of Georgia
          1120 15th St, Augusta, GA  30912
**Phone:** (706) 721-2423
**Fax:** (706) 721-6918
**Percentage of IMGs in the program:** 40%
**Minimum USMLE Step 1 Score Requirement:** 220
**Minimum USMLE Step 2 Score Requirement:** 220
**Attempts on any step:** No limits set
**CS required at time of application:** No

**USCE Requirement:** Yes 6 months
**Cut-Off time since graduation:** 3 years
**Program offers couple match:** Yes
**Visas Sponsored or accepted:** J1 visa

## Emory University Internal Medicine Residency Program

**Specialty:** Internal Medicine
**Program name:** Emory University Program
**Program code:** 140-12-21-105
**State:** Georgia
**Address:** Grady Memorial Hospital
          69 Jesse Hill Jr Dr SE, Atlanta, GA 30303-3219
**Phone:** (404) 251-8778
**Fax:** (404) 525-2957
**Percentage of IMGs in the program:** 8%
**Minimum USMLE Step 1 Score Requirement:** No limits set
**Minimum USMLE Step 2 Score Requirement:** No limits set
**Attempts on any step:** No limits set
**CS required at time of application:** No
**USCE Requirement:** None
**Cut-Off time since graduation:** 5 years unless clinically active
**Program offers couple match:** Yes
**Visas Sponsored or accepted:** J1 visa and H1b visa

# Memorial Health-University Medical Center/Mercer University School of Medicine (Savannah) Internal Medicine Residency Program

**Specialty:** Internal Medicine
**Program name:** Memorial Health-University Medical Center/Mercer University School of Medicine (Savannah) Program
**Program code:** 140-12-12-108
**NRMP Code:** 1971140P0
**Program type:** Community-based university affiliated hospital
**State:** Georgia
**Address:** Memorial University Medical Center
 1101 Lexington Ave, Savannah, GA 31404
**Phone:** (912) 350-7573
**Fax:** (912) 350-7270
**Percentage of IMGs in the program:** 70%
**Minimum USMLE Step 1 Score Requirement:** No limits set
**Minimum USMLE Step 2 Score Requirement:** No limits set
**Attempts on any step:** Must pass on first attempt

**CS required at time of application:** Yes including ECFMG certificate
**USCE Requirement:** None
**Cut-Off time since graduation:** 5 years unless clinically active
**Program offers couple match:** Yes
**Visas Sponsored or accepted:** J1 visa

## Atlanta Medical Center Internal Medicine Residency Program

**Specialty:** Internal Medicine
**Program name:** Atlanta Medical Center Program
**Program code:** 140-12-12-106
**NRMP Code:** 1112140C0
**Program type:** Community-based
**State:** Georgia
**Address:** Atlanta Medical Center,
         303 Parkway Dr NE, Atlanta, GA 30312-1212
**Phone:** (404) 265-4919
**Fax:** (404) 265-4989
**Percentage of IMGs in the program:** 95%
**Minimum USMLE Step 1 Score Requirement:** 210
**Minimum USMLE Step 2 Score Requirement:** 210
**Attempts on any step:** Must pass on first attempt

**CS required at time of application:** Yes
**USCE Requirement:** Yes 1 month
**Cut-Off time since graduation:** 5 years
**Program offers couple match:** Yes
**Visas Sponsored or accepted:** J1 visa

# Hawaii

## University of Hawaii Internal Medicine Residency Program

**Specialty:** Internal Medicine
**Program name:** University of Hawaii Program
**Program code:** 140-14-21-109
**NRMP Code:** 3350140C0, 3350140P0
**Program type:** Community-based university affiliated hospital
**State:** Hawaii
**Address:** University of Hawaii John A Burns School of Medicine
        1356 Lusitana St, Honolulu, HI  96813
**Phone:** (808) 586-2910
**Fax:** (808) 586-7486
**Percentage of IMGs in the program:** 30%
**Minimum USMLE Step 1 Score Requirement:** No limits set

**Minimum USMLE Step 2 Score Requirement:** No limits set
**Attempts on any step:** No limits set
**CS required at time of application:** Yes
**USCE Requirement:** None
**Cut-Off time since graduation:** No limits set
**Program offers couple match:** Yes
**Visas Sponsored or accepted:** J1 visa

# Idaho

## University of Washington (Boise) Internal Medicine Residency Program

**Specialty:** Internal Medicine
**Program name:** University of Washington (Boise) Program
**Program code:** 140-15-12-544
**NRMP Code:** 1172140C0, 1172140P1
**Program type:** Community-based university affiliated hospital
**State:** Idaho
**Address:** Boise VA Medical Center
500 W Fort St, Boise, ID 83702
**Phone:** (208) 422-1314
**Fax:** (208) 422-1388
**Percentage of IMGs in the program:** 5%

**Minimum USMLE Step 1 Score Requirement:**
No limits set
**Minimum USMLE Step 2 Score Requirement:**
No limits set
**Attempts on any step:** No limits set
**CS required at time of application:** Yes
including ECFMG certificate
**USCE Requirement:** Yes 6 months
**Cut-Off time since graduation:** 5 years
**Program offers couple match:** Yes
**Visas Sponsored or accepted:** No visa

# Illinois

## University of Illinois College of Medicine at Peoria Internal Medicine Residency Program

**Specialty:** Internal Medicine
**Program name:** University of Illinois College of
Medicine at Peoria Program
**Program code:** 140-16-31-131
**NRMP Code:** 1175140C0, 1175140P0
**Program type:** Community-based university
affiliated hospital

**State:** Illinois
**Address:** OSF St Francis Medical Center
           530 NE Glen Oak Ave, Peoria, IL  61637
**Phone:** (309) 655-2730
**Percentage of IMGs in the program:** 65%
**Minimum USMLE Step 1 Score Requirement:** 220
**Minimum USMLE Step 2 Score Requirement:** 220
**Attempts on any step:** No limits set
**CS required at time of application:** Yes including ECFMG certificate
**USCE Requirement:** None
**Cut-Off time since graduation:** 5 years unless clinically active
**Program offers couple match:** Yes
**Visas Sponsored or accepted:** J1 visa and H1b visa

## University of Chicago (NorthShore) Internal Medicine Residency Program

**Specialty:** Internal Medicine
**Program name:** University of Chicago (NorthShore) Program
**Program code:** 140-16-31-125
**NRMP Code:** 1160140C2, 1160140P3, 1160140P2
**Program type:** Community-based university

affiliated hospital
**State:** Illinois
**Address:** NorthShore University HealthSystem
2650 Ridge Ave, Evanston, IL  60201
**Phone:** (847) 570-2509
**Fax:** (847) 570-2905
**Percentage of IMGs in the program:** 10%
**Minimum USMLE Step 1 Score Requirement:**
205
**Minimum USMLE Step 2 Score Requirement:**
205
**Attempts on any step:** Must pass on first
attempt including CS exam
**CS required at time of application:** No
**USCE Requirement:** Yes 6 months
**Cut-Off time since graduation:** 5 years
**Program offers couple match:** Yes
**Visas Sponsored or accepted:** J1 visa and H1b
visa


## Mount Sinai Hospital Medical Center of Chicago Internal Medicine Residency Program

**Specialty:** Internal Medicine
**Program name:** Mount Sinai Hospital Medical
Center of Chicago Program
**Program code:** 140-16-21-541

**NRMP Code:** 1144140P0, 1144140C0
**Program type:** Community-based
**State:** Illinois
**Address:** Mount Sinai Hospital Medical Center
1500 S California Ave, Chicago, IL 60608
**Phone:** (773) 257-5077
**Fax:** (773) 257-6027
**Percentage of IMGs in the program:** 70%
**Minimum USMLE Step 1 Score Requirement:** 220
**Minimum USMLE Step 2 Score Requirement:** 220
**Attempts on any step:** Must pass on first attempt including CS exam
**CS required at time of application:** Yes
**USCE Requirement:** None
**Cut-Off time since graduation:** 5 years
**Program offers couple match:** No
**Visas Sponsored or accepted:** J1 visa

## West Suburban Medical Center Internal Medicine Residency Program

**Specialty:** Internal Medicine
**Program name:** West Suburban Medical Center Program
**Program code:** 140-16-21-467

**NRMP Code:** 1173140C0, 1173140P0
**Program type:** Community-based university affiliated hospital
**State:** Illinois
**Address:** West Suburban Medical Center
3 Erie Ct, Oak Park, IL 60302
**Phone:** (708) 763-6908
**Fax:** (708) 763-6655
**Percentage of IMGs in the program:** 90%
**Minimum USMLE Step 1 Score Requirement:** 210
**Minimum USMLE Step 2 Score Requirement:** 210
**Attempts on any step:** Must pass on the first attempt including CS exam
**CS required at time of application:** Yes including ECFMG certificate
**USCE Requirement:** Yes
**Cut-Off time since graduation:** 3 years
**Program offers couple match:** Yes
**Visas Sponsored or accepted:** No visa

## University of Illinois College of Medicine at Urbana Internal Medicine Residency Program

**Specialty:** Internal Medicine
**Program name:** University of Illinois College of Medicine at Urbana Program

**Program code:** 140-16-21-456
**State:** Illinois
**Address:** University of Illinois College of
Medicine Urbana
      611 W Park St, Urbana, IL  61801
**Phone:** (217) 383-3110
**Fax:** (217) 244-0621
**Percentage of IMGs in the program:** 90%
**Minimum USMLE Step 1 Score Requirement:**
205
**Minimum USMLE Step 2 Score Requirement:**
205
**Attempts on any step:** No limits set
**CS required at time of application:** No
**USCE Requirement:** None
**Cut-Off time since graduation:** 5 years unless
clinically active
**Program offers couple match:** Yes
**Visas Sponsored or accepted:** J1 visa and H1b
visa

## Southern Illinois University Internal Medicine Residency Program

**Specialty:** Internal Medicine
**Program name:** Southern Illinois University
Program
**Program code:** 140-16-21-132

**NRMP Code:** 2922140C0, 2922140P0
**Program type:** University-based
**State:** Illinois
**Address:** Southern Illinois University School of Medicine
        701 N First St, Springfield, IL  62794-9636
**Phone:** (217) 545-0193
**Fax:** (217) 545-8156
**Percentage of IMGs in the program:** 70%
**Minimum USMLE Step 1 Score Requirement:** 210
**Minimum USMLE Step 2 Score Requirement:** 210
**Attempts on any step:** Must pass on first attempt including CS exam
**CS required at time of application:** No
**USCE Requirement:** None
**Cut-Off time since graduation:** 3 years
**Program offers couple match:** Yes
**Visas Sponsored or accepted:** J1 visa


# Advocate Lutheran General Hospital Internal Medicine Residency Program

**Specialty:** Internal Medicine
**Program name:** Advocate Lutheran General Hospital Program
**Program code:** 140-16-21-130

**NRMP Code:** 1176140C0, 1176140P0
**Program type:** Community-based university affiliated hospital
**State:** Illinois
**Address:** Advocate Lutheran General Hospital
    1775 W Dempster St, Park Ridge, IL 60068-1174
**Phone:** (847) 723-1680
**Fax:** (847) 723-5615
**Percentage of IMGs in the program:** 20%
**Minimum USMLE Step 1 Score Requirement:** 212
**Minimum USMLE Step 2 Score Requirement:** 212
**Attempts on any step:** Must pass on first attempt
**CS required at time of application:** Yes
**USCE Requirement:** None
**Cut-Off time since graduation:** 3 years
**Program offers couple match:** Yes
**Visas Sponsored or accepted:** No visa

# University of Illinois College of Medicine at Chicago/Advocate Christ Medical Center Internal Medicine Residency Program

**Specialty:** Internal Medicine

**Program name:** University of Illinois College of Medicine at Chicago/Advocate Christ Medical Center Program
**Program code:** 140-16-21-129
**NRMP Code:** 1150140P1, 1150140C0
**Program type:** Community-based university affiliated hospital
**State:** Illinois
**Address:** Advocate Christ Medical Center
4440 W 95th St, Oak Lawn, IL  60453
**Phone:** (708) 684-5673
**Fax:** (708) 684-2500
**Percentage of IMGs in the program:** 80%
**Minimum USMLE Step 1 Score Requirement:** 205
**Minimum USMLE Step 2 Score Requirement:** 205
**Attempts on any step:** No limits set
**CS required at time of application:** No
**USCE Requirement:** Yes
**Cut-Off time since graduation:** 3 years
**Program offers couple match:** Yes
**Visas Sponsored or accepted:** J1 visa

## Loyola University Internal Medicine Residency Program

**Specialty:** Internal Medicine
**Program name:** Loyola University Program
**Program code:** 140-16-21-128

**NRMP Code:** 1170140C0, 1170140P0
**Program type:** University-based
**State:** Illinois
**Address:** Loyola University Medical Center
2160 S First Ave, Maywood, IL 60153
**Phone:** (708) 216-6053
**Fax:** (708) 216-6890
**Percentage of IMGs in the program:** 8%
**Minimum USMLE Step 1 Score Requirement:** 205
**Minimum USMLE Step 2 Score Requirement:** 205
**Attempts on any step:** No limits set
**CS required at time of application:** Yes including ECFMG certificate
**USCE Requirement:** None
**Cut-Off time since graduation:** 4 years
**Program offers couple match:** Yes
**Visas Sponsored or accepted:** J1 visa

# Chicago Medical School at Rosalind Franklin University of Medicine and Science Internal Medicine Residency Program

**Specialty:** Internal Medicine
**Program name:** Chicago Medical School at Rosalind Franklin University of Medicine and Science Program

**Program code:** 140-16-21-111
**NRMP Code:** 3053140C0
**Program type:** University-based
**State:** Illinois
**Address:** Rosalind Franklin University/Chicago Medical School

3333 Green Bay Rd, North Chicago, IL 60064-3095
**Phone:** (847) 578-3227
**Fax:** (847) 578-8647
**Percentage of IMGs in the program:** 100%
**Minimum USMLE Step 1 Score Requirement:** 205
**Minimum USMLE Step 2 Score Requirement:** 205
**Attempts on any step:** Must pass on first attempt on any step including CS exam
**CS required at time of application:** Yes
**USCE Requirement:** Yes 1 month
**Cut-Off time since graduation:** 5 years unless clinically active
**Program offers couple match:** No
**Visas Sponsored or accepted:** J1 visa


## John H Stroger Hospital of Cook County Internal Medicine Residency Program

**Specialty:** Internal Medicine

**Program name:** John H Stroger Hospital of Cook County Program
**Program code:** 140-16-12-113
**NRMP Code:** 1127140C0, 1127140M0,
**Program type:** Community-based university affiliated hospital
**State:** Illinois
**Address:** Stroger Hospital of Cook County
          1900 W Polk St, Chicago, IL  60612
**Phone:** (312) 864-7229
**Fax:** (312) 864-9725
**Percentage of IMGs in the program:** 60%
**Minimum USMLE Step 1 Score Requirement:** 220
**Minimum USMLE Step 2 Score Requirement:** 220
**Attempts on any step:** Must pass on first attempt including CS exam
**CS required at time of application:** No
**USCE Requirement:** None
**Cut-Off time since graduation:** 5 years
**Program offers couple match:** Yes
**Visas Sponsored or accepted:** J1 visa and H1b visa

## MacNeal Hospital Internal Medicine Residency Program

**Specialty:** Internal Medicine
**Program name:** MacNeal Hospital Program

**Program code:** 140-16-11-454
**NRMP Code:** 1121140C0
**Program type:** Community-based university affiliated hospital
**State:** Illinois
**Address:** MacNeal Hospital
          3249 S Oak Park Ave, Berwyn, IL 60402
**Phone:** (708) 783-3401
**Fax:** (708) 783-3341
**Percentage of IMGs in the program:** 100%
**Minimum USMLE Step 1 Score Requirement:** 205
**Minimum USMLE Step 2 Score Requirement:** 205
**Attempts on any step:** No limits set
**CS required at time of application:** Yes
**USCE Requirement:** Yes
**Cut-Off time since graduation:** 5 years unless clinically active
**Program offers couple match:** No
**Visas Sponsored or accepted:** J1 visa


## Presence St Francis Hospital Internal Medicine Residency Program

**Specialty:** Internal Medicine
**Program name:** Presence St Francis Hospital Program

(Old Name: St Francis Hospital of Evanston Program)
**Program code:** 140-16-11-126
**NRMP Code:** 1168140C0, 1168140P0
**Program type:** Community-based university affiliated hospital
**State:** Illinois
**Address:** St Francis Hospital
355 Ridge Ave, Evanston, IL  60202-3399
**Phone:** (847) 316-6228
**Fax:** (847) 316-3307
**Percentage of IMGs in the program:** 80%
**Minimum USMLE Step 1 Score Requirement:** 220
**Minimum USMLE Step 2 Score Requirement:** 220
**Attempts on any step:** Must pass on first attempt
**CS required at time of application:** Yes
**USCE Requirement:** None
**Cut-Off time since graduation:** 5 years unless clinically active
**Program offers couple match:** Yes
**Visas Sponsored or accepted:** J1 visa and H1b visa

# Presence St Joseph Hospital (Chicago) Internal Medicine Residency Program

**Specialty:** Internal Medicine
**Program name:** Presence St Joseph Hospital (Chicago) Program
**Program code:** 140-16-11-122
**State:** Illinois
**Address:** St Joseph Hospital
            2900 N Lake Shore Dr, Chicago, IL 60657
**Phone:** (773) 665-3022
**Fax:** (773) 665-3384
**Percentage of IMGs in the program:** 90%
**Minimum USMLE Step 1 Score Requirement:** 205
**Minimum USMLE Step 2 Score Requirement:** 205
**Attempts on any step:** Must pass from maximum on 2nd attempt including CS exam
**CS required at time of application:** Yes
**USCE Requirement:** None
**Cut-Off time since graduation:** 5 years unless clinically active
**Program offers couple match:** Yes
**Visas Sponsored or accepted:** J1 visa and H1b visa

# Rush University Medical Center Internal Medicine Residency Program

**Specialty:** Internal Medicine
**Program name:** Rush University Medical Center Program
**Program code:** 140-16-11-121
**NRMP Code:** 1147140C0, 1147140P1, 1147140P0
**Program type:** University-based
**State:** Illinois
**Address:** Rush University Medical Center
1653 W Congress Pkwy, Chicago, IL 60612
**Phone**: (312) 942-5352
**Fax:** (312) 942-5271
**Percentage of IMGs in the program:** 10%
**Minimum USMLE Step 1 Score Requirement:** 220
**Minimum USMLE Step 2 Score Requirement:** 220
**Attempts on any step:** Must pass on first attempt
**CS required at time of application:** No
**USCE Requirement:** None
**Cut-Off time since graduation:** 4 years
**Program offers couple match:** Yes
**Visas Sponsored or accepted:** J1 visa and H1b visa

# Mercy Hospital and Medical Center Internal Medicine Residency Program

**Specialty:** Internal Medicine
**Program name:** Mercy Hospital and Medical Center Program
**Program code:** 140-16-11-116
**State:** Illinois
**Address:** Mercy Hospital and Medical Center
        2525 S Michigan Ave, Chicago, IL 60616-2477
**Phone:** (312) 567-2053
**Fax:** (312) 567-2695
**Percentage of IMGs in the program:** 90%
**Minimum USMLE Step 1 Score Requirement:** 205
**Minimum USMLE Step 2 Score Requirement:** 205
**Attempts on any step:** Maximum of 2 attempts allowed on any step
**CS required at time of application:** No
**USCE Requirement:** Yes
**Cut-Off time since graduation:** 5 years
**Program offers couple match:** Yes
**Visas Sponsored or accepted:** J1 visa

# Louis A Weiss Memorial Hospital Internal Medicine Residency Program

**Specialty:** Internal Medicine
**Program name:** Louis A Weiss Memorial Hospital Program
**Program code:** 140-16-11-115
**NRMP Code:** 1846140P0, 1846140C0
**Program type:** Community-based university affiliated hospital
**State:** Illinois
**Address:** Louis A Weiss Memorial Hospital
4646 N Marine Dr, Chicago, IL  60640
**Phone:** (773) 564-7294
**Fax:** (773) 564-5226
**Percentage of IMGs in the program:** 70%
**Minimum USMLE Step 1 Score Requirement:** 225
**Minimum USMLE Step 2 Score Requirement:** 225
**Attempts on any step:** No limits set
**CS required at time of application:** No
**USCE Requirement:** None
**Cut-Off time since graduation:** No limits set
**Program offers couple match:** No
**Visas Sponsored or accepted:** J1 visa

## Advocate Illinois Masonic Medical Center/North Side Health Network Internal Medicine Residency Program

**Specialty:** Internal Medicine
**Program name:** Advocate Illinois Masonic Medical Center/North Side Health Network Program
**Program code:** 140-16-11-114
**NRMP Code:** 1137140P0, 1137140C0
**Program type:** Community-based university affiliated hospital
**State:** Illinois
**Address:** Advocate Illinois Masonic Medical Center
836 W Wellington Ave, Chicago, IL 60657-5193
**Phone:** (773) 296-7635
**Fax:** (773) 296-7486
**Percentage of IMGs in the program:** 80%
**Minimum USMLE Step 1 Score Requirement:** 215
**Minimum USMLE Step 2 Score Requirement:** 215
**Attempts on any step:** No limits set
**CS required at time of application:** No
**USCE Requirement:** None
**Cut-Off time since graduation:** 5 years
**Program offers couple match:** Yes

**Visas Sponsored or accepted:** J1 visa

# Indiana

## Indiana University School of Medicine Internal Medicine Residency Program

**Specialty:** Internal Medicine
**Program name:** Indiana University School of Medicine Program
**Program code:** 140-17-21-133
**NRMP Code:** 1187140C0
**Program type:** University-based
**State:** Indiana
**Address:** Wishard Memorial Hospital
1001 W 10th St, Indianapolis, IN 46202
**Phone:** (317) 656-4276
**Fax:** (317) 630-2667
**Percentage of IMGs in the program:** 20%
**Minimum USMLE Step 1 Score Requirement:** 215
**Minimum USMLE Step 2 Score Requirement:** 215
**Attempts on any step:** Must pass on first attempt
**CS required at time of application:** No
**USCE Requirement:** Yes

**Cut-Off time since graduation:** 3 years
**Program offers couple match:** Yes
**Visas Sponsored or accepted:** J1 visa

## Indiana University Health Ball Memorial Hospital Internal Medicine Residency Program

**Specialty:** Internal Medicine
**Program name:** Indiana University Health Ball Memorial Hospital Program
**Program code:** 140-17-11-136
**NRMP Code:** 1192140C0
**Program type:** Community-based university affiliated hospital
**State:** Indiana
**Address:** IU Health Ball Memorial Hospital
2401 W University Ave, Muncie, IN 47303
**Phone:** (765) 747-3367
**Fax:** (765) 751-1451
**Percentage of IMGs in the program:** 70%
**Minimum USMLE Step 1 Score Requirement:** No limits set
**Minimum USMLE Step 2 Score Requirement:** No limits set
**Attempts on any step:** No limits set
**CS required at time of application:** No
**USCE Requirement:** None

**Cut-Off time since graduation:** 5 years unless clinically active
**Program offers couple match:** Yes
**Visas Sponsored or accepted:** J1 visa and H1b visa

## St Vincent Hospitals and Health Care Center Internal Medicine Residency Program

**Specialty:** Internal Medicine
**Program name:** St Vincent Hospitals and Health Care Center Program
**Program code:** 140-17-11-135
**NRMP Code:** 1189140M0, 1189140P0, 1189140C0
**Program type:** Community-based university affiliated hospital
**State:** Indiana
**Address:** St Vincent Hosp and Health Care Center
        2001 W 86th St, Indianapolis, IN 46260
**Phone:** (317) 338-2564
**Fax:** (317) 338-6359
**Percentage of IMGs in the program:** 20%
**Minimum USMLE Step 1 Score Requirement:** 205
**Minimum USMLE Step 2 Score Requirement:** 205

**Attempts on any step:** Must pass on first attempt including CS exam
**CS required at time of application:** No
**USCE Requirement:** Yes 3 months
**Cut-Off time since graduation:** 5 years
**Program offers couple match:** Yes
**Visas Sponsored or accepted:** J1 visa

# Iowa

## University of Iowa (Des Moines) Internal Medicine Residency Program

**Specialty:** Internal Medicine
**Program name:** University of Iowa (Des Moines) Program
**Program code:** 140-18-31-137
**NRMP Code:** 1201140C0, 1201140P0
**Program type:** Community-based university affiliated hospital
**State:** Iowa
**Address:** Iowa Methodist Medical Center
        1415 Woodland Ave, Des Moines, IA 50309
**Phone:** (515) 241-5995

**Fax:** (515) 241-6576
**Percentage of IMGs in the program:** 15%
**Minimum USMLE Step 1 Score Requirement:**
205
**Minimum USMLE Step 2 Score Requirement:**
205
**Attempts on any step:** Must pass on first
attempt including CS exam
**CS required at time of application:** No
**USCE Requirement:** Yes 3 months
**Cut-Off time since graduation:** 5 years
**Program offers couple match:** Yes
**Visas Sponsored or accepted:** J1 visa


# University of Iowa Hospitals and Clinics Internal Medicine Residency Program

**Specialty:** Internal Medicine
**Program name:** University of Iowa Hospitals
and Clinics Program
**Program code:** 140-18-21-138
**NRMP Code:** 1203140P1, 1203140P0,
1203140C0
**Program type:** University-based
**State:** Iowa
**Address:** University of Iowa Hospitals and
Clinics
          200 Hawkins Dr, Iowa City, IA  52242-

1081
**Phone:** (319) 356-2034
**Fax:** (319) 384-8955
**Percentage of IMGs in the program:** 25%
**Minimum USMLE Step 1 Score Requirement:**
No limits set
**Minimum USMLE Step 2 Score Requirement:**
No limits set
**Attempts on any step:** Must pass on first
attempt including CS exam
**CS required at time of application:** No
**USCE Requirement:** Yes 1 month
**Cut-Off time since graduation:** No limits set
**Program offers couple match:** Yes
**Visas Sponsored or accepted:** J1 visa and H1b
visa

# Kansas

## University of Kansas School of Medicine Internal Medicine Residency Program

**Specialty:** Internal Medicine
**Program name:** University of Kansas School of
Medicine Program
**Program code:** 140-19-21-139

**NRMP Code:** University of Kansas Hospital and Medical Center
**Program type:** University-based
**State:** Kansas
**Address:** University of Kansas Medical Center
3901 Rainbow Blvd, Kansas City, KS 66160-7350
**Phone:** (913) 945-7072
**Fax:** (913) 588-0890
**Percentage of IMGs in the program:** 30%
**Minimum USMLE Step 1 Score Requirement:** 220
**Minimum USMLE Step 2 Score Requirement:** 220
**Attempts on any step:** Must pass on first attempt including CS exam
**CS required at time of application:** No
**USCE Requirement:** None
**Cut-Off time since graduation:** 5 years
**Program offers couple match:** Yes
**Visas Sponsored or accepted:** J1 visa

## University of Kansas (Wichita) Internal Medicine Residency Program

**Specialty:** Internal Medicine
**Program name:** University of Kansas (Wichita) Program
**Program code:** 140-19-21-140

**NRMP Code:** 3054140C0, 3054140P0
**Program type:** Community-based university affiliated hospital
**State:** Kansas
**Address:** University of Kansas School of Medicine-Wichita
     1010 N Kansas, Wichita, KS  67214-3799
**Phone:** (316) 293-2650
**Fax:** (316) 293-1878
**Percentage of IMGs in the program:** 55%
**Minimum USMLE Step 1 Score Requirement:** No limits set
**Minimum USMLE Step 2 Score Requirement:** No limits set
**Attempts on any step:** No limits set
**CS required at time of application:** Yes
**USCE Requirement:** None
**Cut-Off time since graduation:** No limits set
**Program offers couple match:** Yes
**Visas Sponsored or accepted:** J1 visa


# Kentucky

## University of Louisville Internal Medicine Residency Program

**Specialty:** Internal Medicine
**Program name:** University of Louisville Program
**Program code:** 140-20-31-142
**NRMP Code:** 1217140C0, 1217140P0
**Program type:** University-based
**State:** Kentucky
**Address:** University of Louisville Hospital
550 S Jackson St, Louisville, KY  40202
**Phone:** (502) 852-7041
**Fax:** (502) 852-8980
**Percentage of IMGs in the program:** 20%
**Minimum USMLE Step 1 Score Requirement:** 220
**Minimum USMLE Step 2 Score Requirement:** 220
**Attempts on any step:** No limits set
**CS required at time of application:** No
**USCE Requirement:** None
**Cut-Off time since graduation:** 3 years
**Program offers couple match:** Yes
**Visas Sponsored or accepted:** J1 visa


## University of  Kentucky College of Medicine Internal Medicine Residency Program

**Specialty:** Internal Medicine
**Program name:** University of Kentucky College of Medicine Program
**Program code:** 140-20-21-141
**NRMP Code:** 1848140C0, 1848140M0, 1848140P0
**Program type:** University-based
**State:** Kentucky
**Address:** University of Kentucky-Chandler Medical Center
            900 S Limestone St, Lexington, KY 40536-0200
**Phone:** (859) 323-9918
**Fax:** (859) 323-1197
**Percentage of IMGs in the program:** 35%
**Minimum USMLE Step 1 Score Requirement:** No limits set
**Minimum USMLE Step 2 Score Requirement:** No limits set
**Attempts on any step:** Must pass maximum on 2nd attempt including CS exam
**CS required at time of application:** Yes
**USCE Requirement:** None
**Cut-Off time since graduation:** 4 years unless clinically active
**Program offers couple match:** Yes
**Visas Sponsored or accepted:** J1 visa

# Louisiana

## Baton Rouge General Medical Center Internal Medicine Residency Program

**Specialty:** Internal Medicine
**Program name:** Baton Rouge General Medical Center Program
**Program code:** 140-21-31-543
**NRMP Code:** 1139140C0
**Program type:** Community-based university affiliated hospital
**State:** Louisiana
**Address:** Baton Rouge General Medical Center
3600 Florida Blvd, Baton Rouge, LA 70806
**Phone:** (225) 381-6762
**Fax:** (225) 387-7872
**Percentage of IMGs in the program:** 40%
**Minimum USMLE Step 1 Score Requirement:** No limits set
**Minimum USMLE Step 2 Score Requirement:** No limits set
**Attempts on any step:** No limits set
**CS required at time of application:** Yes
**USCE Requirement:** None
**Cut-Off time since graduation:** 3 years
**Program offers couple match:** Yes
**Visas Sponsored or accepted:** No visa

## Ochsner Clinic Foundation Internal Medicine Residency Program

**Specialty:** Internal Medicine
**Program name:** Ochsner Clinic Foundation Program
**Program code:** 140-21-22-146
**NRMP Code:** 1966140P0, 1966140C0
**Program type:** Community-based
**State:** Louisiana
**Address:** Ochsner Clinic Foundation
            1514 Jefferson Hwy, New Orleans, LA 70121
**Phone:** (504) 842-0450
**Fax:** (504) 842-3327
**Percentage of IMGs in the program:** 30%
**Minimum USMLE Step 1 Score Requirement:** 210
**Minimum USMLE Step 2 Score Requirement:** 210
**Attempts on any step:** Must pass maximum on 2nd attempt including CS exam
**CS required at time of application:** Yes including ECFMG certificate
**USCE Requirement:** Yes 1 month
**Cut-Off time since graduation:** 3 years
**Program offers couple match:** Yes
**Visas Sponsored or accepted:** J1 visa

# Leonard J Chabert Medical Center Internal Medicine Residency Program

**Specialty:** Internal Medicine
**Program name:** Leonard J Chabert Medical Center Program
**Program code:** 140-21-21-537
**State:** Louisiana
**Address:** Leonard J Chabert Medical Center
           1978 Industrial Blvd, Houma, LA 70363
**Phone:** (985) 873-2710
**Fax:** (985) 873-2722
**Percentage of IMGs in the program:** 95%
**Minimum USMLE Step 1 Score Requirement:** No limits set
**Minimum USMLE Step 2 Score Requirement:** No limits set
**Attempts on any step:** Must pass on first attempt including CS exam
**CS required at time of application:** Yes
**USCE Requirement:** None
**Cut-Off time since graduation:** 2 years
**Program offers couple match:** Yes
**Visas Sponsored or accepted:** J1 visa

# Louisiana State University (Shreveport) Internal Medicine Residency Program

**Specialty:** Internal Medicine
**Program name:** Louisiana State University (Shreveport) Program
**Program code:** 140-21-21-148
**NRMP Code:** 1232140M0, 1232140C0, 1232140P0
**Program type:** University-based
**State:** Louisiana
**Address:** LSU Health Sciences Center Shreveport,
          1501 Kings Highway, Shreveport, LA 71130-3932
**Phone:** (318) 675-4314
**Fax:** (318) 675-5958
**Percentage of IMGs in the program:** 70%
**Minimum USMLE Step 1 Score Requirement:** 210
**Minimum USMLE Step 2 Score Requirement:** 210
**Attempts on any step:** Must pass on first attempt including CS exam
**CS required at time of application:** No
**USCE Requirement:** Yes
**Cut-Off time since graduation:** No limits set
**Program offers couple match:** Yes
**Visas Sponsored or accepted:** J1 visa

# Louisiana State University Internal Medicine Residency Program

**Specialty:** Internal Medicine
**Program name:** Louisiana State University Program
**Program code:** 140-21-21-143
**NRMP Code:** 1224140C0, 1224140P0
**Program type:** University-based
**State:** Louisiana
**Address:** Louisiana State University Health Science Center New Orleans
          1542 Tulane Ave, New Orleans, LA 70112
**Phone:** (504) 568-5600
**Fax:** (504) 568-7884
**Percentage of IMGs in the program:** 5%
**Minimum USMLE Step 1 Score Requirement:** 220
**Minimum USMLE Step 2 Score Requirement:** 220
**Attempts on any step:** No limits set
**CS required at time of application:** No
**USCE Requirement:** None
**Cut-Off time since graduation:** 2 years
**Program offers couple match:** Yes
**Visas Sponsored or accepted:** J1 visa

# University Medical Center/Louisiana State University (Lafayette) Internal Medicine Residency Program

**Specialty:** Internal Medicine
**Program name:** University Medical Center/Louisiana State University (Lafayette) Program
**Program code:** 140-21-11-144
**NRMP Code:** 1225140C0, 1225140P0
**Program type:** Community-based university affiliated hospital
**State:** Louisiana
**Address:** University Hospital and Clinics
2390 W Congress St, Lafayette, LA 70506
**Phone:** (337) 261-6789
**Fax:** (337) 261-6791
**Percentage of IMGs in the program:** 70%
**Minimum USMLE Step 1 Score Requirement:** 220
**Minimum USMLE Step 2 Score Requirement:** 220
**Attempts on any step:** Must pass on maximum 2nd attempt including CS exam
**CS required at time of application:** Yes including ECFMG certificate
**USCE Requirement:** None
**Cut-Off time since graduation:** No limits set

**Program offers couple match:** Yes
**Visas Sponsored or accepted:** J1 visa

## Maine

### Maine Medical Center Internal Medicine Residency Program

**Specialty:** Internal Medicine
**Program name:** Maine Medical Center Program
**Program code:** 140-22-11-149
**NRMP Code:** 1236140C0
**Program type:** Community-based university affiliated hospital
**State:** Maine
**Address:** Maine Medical Center
22 Bramhall St, Portland, ME 04102
**Phone:** (207) 662-2651
**Fax:** (207) 662-6788
**Percentage of IMGs in the program:** 5%
**Minimum USMLE Step 1 Score Requirement:** 205
**Minimum USMLE Step 2 Score Requirement:** 205
**Attempts on any step:** No limits set
**CS required at time of application:** Yes including ECFMG certificate
**USCE Requirement:** Yes 6 months

**Cut-Off time since graduation:** 5 years
**Program offers couple match:** Yes
**Visas Sponsored or accepted:** J1 visa

## Maryland

### Harbor Hospital Center Internal Medicine Residency Program

**Specialty:** Internal Medicine
**Program name:** Harbor Hospital Center Program
**Program code:** 140-23-31-158
**NRMP Code:** 1250140C0, 1250140P0
**Program type:** Community-based
**State:** Maryland
**Address:** MedStar Harbor Hospital
3001 S Hanover St, Baltimore, MD 21225-1290
**Phone:** (410) 350-3565
**Fax:** (410) 354-0186
**Percentage of IMGs in the program:** 60%
**Minimum USMLE Step 1 Score Requirement:** 240
**Minimum USMLE Step 2 Score Requirement:** 240

**Attempts on any step:** Must pass on first attempt
**CS required at time of application:** Yes
**USCE Requirement:** None
**Cut-Off time since graduation:** No limits set
**Program offers couple match:** Yes
**Visas Sponsored or accepted:** J1 visa and H1b visa

## Greater Baltimore Medical Center Internal Medicine Residency Program

**Specialty:** Internal Medicine
**Program name:** Greater Baltimore Medical Center Program
**Program code:** 140-23-31-152
**NRMP Code:** 1241140P0, 1241140M0
**Program type:** Community-based
**State:** Maryland
**Address:** Greater Baltimore Medical Center
6565 N Charles St, Towson, MD  21204
**Phone:** (443) 849-2682
**Fax:** (443) 849-8030
**Percentage of IMGs in the program:** 80%
**Minimum USMLE Step 1 Score Requirement:** 230
**Minimum USMLE Step 2 Score Requirement:** 230

**Attempts on any step:** Must pass on first attempt including CS exam
**CS required at time of application:** Yes
**USCE Requirement:** None
**Cut-Off time since graduation:** No limits set
**Program offers couple match:** Yes
**Visas Sponsored or accepted:** J1 visa

## Good Samaritan Hospital of Maryland Internal Medicine Residency Program

**Specialty:** Internal Medicine
**Program name:** Good Samaritan Hospital of Maryland Program
**Program code:** 140-23-21-489
**State:** Maryland
**Address:** Good Samaritan Hospital,
            5601 Loch Raven Blvd, Baltimore, MD 21239
**Phone:** (443) 444-4863
**Fax:** (443) 444-4997
**Percentage of IMGs in the program:** 100%
**Minimum USMLE Step 1 Score Requirement:** 225
**Minimum USMLE Step 2 Score Requirement:** 225
**Attempts on any step:** No limits set
**CS required at time of application:** Yes including ECFMG certificate

**USCE Requirement:** None
**Cut-Off time since graduation:** 10 years
**Program offers couple match:** Yes
**Visas Sponsored or accepted:** J1 visa and H1b visa

## Prince George's Hospital Center Internal Medicine Residency Program

**Specialty:** Internal Medicine
**Program name:** Prince George's Hospital Center Program
**Program code:** 140-23-21-161
**NRMP Code:** 1905140C0, 1905140P0
**Program type:** Community-based
**State:** Maryland
**Address:** Prince George's Hospital Center
      3001 Hospital Dr, Cheverly, MD 20785
**Phone:** (301) 618-3772
**Fax:** (301) 618-2986
**Percentage of IMGs in the program:** 100%
**Minimum USMLE Step 1 Score Requirement:** 207
**Minimum USMLE Step 2 Score Requirement:** 207
**Attempts on any step:** Must pass maximum on 2nd attempt
**CS required at time of application:** Yes including ECFMG certificate

**USCE Requirement:** None
**Cut-Off time since graduation:** 10 years
**Program offers couple match:** No
**Visas Sponsored or accepted:** J1 visa and H1b visa

## Sinai Hospital of Baltimore Internal Medicine Residency Program

**Specialty:** Internal Medicine
**Program name:** Sinai Hospital of Baltimore Program
**Program code:** 140-23-12-157
**NRMP Code:** 1893140P0, 1893140C0
**Program type:** Community-based university affiliated hospital
**State:** Maryland
**Address:** Sinai Hospital of Baltimore
        2435 W Belvedere Ave, Baltimore, MD 21215
**Phone:** (410) 601-7068
**Fax:** (410) 601-7245
**Percentage of IMGs in the program:** 75%
**Minimum USMLE Step 1 Score Requirement:** 210
**Minimum USMLE Step 2 Score Requirement:** 210
**Attempts on any step:** Must pass on first attempt including CS exam
**CS required at time of application:** Yes

**USCE Requirement:** None
**Cut-Off time since graduation:** 5 years
**Program offers couple match:** No
**Visas Sponsored or accepted:** J1 visa

## MedStar Union Memorial Hospital Internal Medicine Residency Program

**Specialty:** Internal Medicine
**Program name:** MedStar Union Memorial Hospital Program
**Program code:** 140-23-12-159
**NRMP Code:** 1251140P0, 1251140C0
**Program type:** Community-based
**State:** Maryland
**Address:** Union Memorial Hospital
          201 E University Pkwy, Baltimore, MD 21218-2895
**Phone:** (410) 554-2060
**Fax:** (410) 554-2184
**Percentage of IMGs in the program:** 75%
**Minimum USMLE Step 1 Score Requirement:** 210
**Minimum USMLE Step 2 Score Requirement:** 210
**Attempts on any step:** Must pass on first attempt
**CS required at time of application:** Yes
**USCE Requirement:** Yes 3 months

**Cut-Off time since graduation:** 3 years
**Program offers couple match:** Yes
**Visas Sponsored or accepted:** J1 visa and H1b visa

## MedStar Franklin Square Hospital Center Internal Medicine Residency Program

**Specialty:** Internal Medicine
**Program name:** MedStar Franklin Square Hospital Center Program
**Program code:** 140-23-12-151
**NRMP Code:** 1240140P0, 1240140C0
**Program type:** Community-based university affiliated hospital
**State:** Maryland
**Address:** MedStar Franklin Square Medical Center
            9000 Franklin Square Dr, Baltimore, MD  21237-3998
**Phone:** (800) 688-8169
**Fax:** (443) 777-8155
**Percentage of IMGs in the program:** 70%
**Minimum USMLE Step 1 Score Requirement:** 205
**Minimum USMLE Step 2 Score Requirement:** 205
**Attempts on any step:** Must pass on first attempt

**CS required at time of application:** No
**USCE Requirement:** None, however 4 months of post Medical school experience in any country is required.
**Cut-Off time since graduation:** 7 years
**Program offers couple match:** Yes
**Visas Sponsored or accepted:** J1 visa

## St Agnes HealthCare Internal Medicine Residency Program

**Specialty:** Internal Medicine
**Program name:** St Agnes HealthCare Program
**Program code:** 140-23-12-156
**NRMP Code:** 1247140P0
**Program type:** Community-based
**State:** Maryland
**Address:** St Agnes Hospital
900 Caton Ave, Baltimore, MD  21229
**Phone:** (410) 368-8858
**Fax:** (410) 368-3525
**Percentage of IMGs in the program:** 100%
**Minimum USMLE Step 1 Score Requirement:** 220
**Minimum USMLE Step 2 Score Requirement:** 220
**Attempts on any step:** Must pass on first attempt including CS exam
**CS required at time of application:** Yes including ECFMG certificate

**USCE Requirement:** Yes 3 months
**Cut-Off time since graduation:** 5 years
**Program offers couple match:** Yes
**Visas Sponsored or accepted:** J1 visa and H1b visa

## University of Maryland Medical Center Midtown Campus Internal Medicine Residency Program

**Specialty:** Internal Medicine
**Program name:** University of Maryland Medical Center Midtown Campus Program
　　　(Old Name: Maryland General Hospital Program)
**Program code:** 140-23-11-154
**State:** Maryland
**Address:** University of Maryland Medical Center
　　　827 Linden Ave, Baltimore, MD 21201
**Phone:** (410) 225-8790
**Fax:** (410) 225-8910
**Percentage of IMGs in the program:** 50%
**Minimum USMLE Step 1 Score Requirement:** 210
**Minimum USMLE Step 2 Score Requirement:** 210
**Attempts on any step:** Must pass on first attempt

**CS required at time of application:** Yes including ECFMG certificate
**USCE Requirement:** None
**Cut-Off time since graduation:** 5 years
**Program offers couple match:** No
**Visas Sponsored or accepted:** J1 visa

## Massachusetts

### Steward Carney Hospital Internal Medicine Residency Program

**Specialty:** Internal Medicine
**Program name:** Steward Carney Hospital Program
**Program code:** 140-24-11-166
**State:** Massachusetts
**Address:** Carney Hospital, Department of Medicine,
        2100 Dorchester Ave, Boston, MA 02124-5666
**Phone:** (617) 506-2726
**Fax:** (617) 506-2110
**Percentage of IMGs in the program:** 20%
**Minimum USMLE Step 1 Score Requirement:** 220
**Minimum USMLE Step 2 Score Requirement:** 220

**Attempts on any step:** Must pass on first attempt
**CS required at time of application:** Yes including ECFMG certificate
**USCE Requirement:** Yes 1 month
**Cut-Off time since graduation:** 5 years
**Program offers couple match:** Yes
**Visas Sponsored or accepted:** J1 visa

## Mount Auburn Hospital Internal Medicine Residency Program

**Specialty:** Internal Medicine
**Program name:** Mount Auburn Hospital Program
**Program code:** 140-24-11-176
**NRMP Code:** 1269140C0, 1269140P0
**Program type:** Community-based university affiliated hospital
**State:** Massachusetts
**Address:** Mount Auburn Hospital, Department of Medicine,
          330 Mount Auburn St, Cambridge, MA  02138
**Phone:** (617) 499-5571
**Fax:** (617) 499-5593
**Percentage of IMGs in the program:** 40%
**Minimum USMLE Step 1 Score Requirement:** No limits set

**Minimum USMLE Step 2 Score Requirement:** No limits set
**Attempts on any step:** No limits set
**CS required at time of application:** Yes including ECFMG certificate
**USCE Requirement:** None
**Cut-Off time since graduation:** No limits set
**Program offers couple match:** Yes
**Visas Sponsored or accepted:** J1 visa and H1b visa

## Berkshire Medical Center Internal Medicine Residency Program

**Specialty:** Internal Medicine
**Program name:** Berkshire Medical Center Program
**Program code:** 140-24-11-179
**NRMP Code:** 1281140C0, 1281140P0
**Program type:** Community-based university affiliated hospital
**State:** Massachusetts
**Address:** Berkshire Medical Center, Department of Internal Medicine,
        725 North St, Pittsfield, MA  01201
**Phone:** (413) 447-2839
**Fax:** (413) 447-2088
**Percentage of IMGs in the program:** 80%
**Minimum USMLE Step 1 Score Requirement:** 210

**Minimum USMLE Step 2 Score Requirement:** 210
**Attempts on any step:** No limits set
**CS required at time of application:** Yes
**USCE Requirement:** None
**Cut-Off time since graduation:** 10 years
**Program offers couple match:** Yes
**Visas Sponsored or accepted:** J1 visa and H1b visa

## Baystate Medical Center/Tufts University School of Medicine Internal Medicine Residency Program

**Specialty:** Internal Medicine
**Program name:** Baystate Medical Center/Tufts University School of Medicine Program
**Program code:** 140-24-11-181
**NRMP Code:** 1286140M0, 1286140C0, 1286140P0
**Program type:** Community-based university affiliated hospital
**State:** Massachusetts
**Address:** Baystate Medical Center, Department of Medicine,
           759 Chestnut St, Springfield, MA 01199
**Phone:** (413) 794-4143
**Fax:** (413) 794-8075

**Percentage of IMGs in the program:** 60%
**Minimum USMLE Step 1 Score Requirement:** No limits set
**Minimum USMLE Step 2 Score Requirement:** No limits set
**Attempts on any step:** Must pass on first attempt
**CS required at time of application:** Yes including ECFMG certificate
**USCE Requirement:** None
**Cut-Off time since graduation:** 3 years during which you should be clinically active
**Program offers couple match:** Yes
**Visas Sponsored or accepted:** J1 visa (H1b visa for select candidates)

## St Vincent Hospital Internal Medicine Residency Program

**Specialty:** Internal Medicine
**Program name:** St Vincent Hospital Program
**Program code:** 140-24-11-183
**NRMP Code:** 1290140C0, 1290140P0
**Program type:** Community-based university affiliated hospital
**State:** Massachusetts
**Address:** St Vincent Hospital, Department of Medicine,
        123 Summer St, Worcester, MA 01608-1320

**Phone:** (508) 363-6208
**Fax:** (508) 363-9798
**Percentage of IMGs in the program:** 60%
**Minimum USMLE Step 1 Score Requirement:** No limits set
**Minimum USMLE Step 2 Score Requirement:** No limits set
**Attempts on any step:** No limits set
**CS required at time of application:** Yes including ECFMG certificate
**USCE Requirement:** None
**Cut-Off time since graduation:** Must be clinically active if graduated more than 2 years
**Program offers couple match:** Yes
**Visas Sponsored or accepted:** J1 visa

## Salem Hospital Internal Medicine Residency Program

**Specialty:** Internal Medicine
**Program name:** Salem Hospital Program
**Program code:** 140-24-12-180
**NRMP Code:** Community-based university affiliated hospital
**Program type:** 1284140C0, 1284140P1, 1284140P0
**State:** Massachusetts
**Address:** Salem Hospital, Suite 317,
          79 Highland Ave, Salem, MA  01970
**Phone:** (978) 354-4021

**Percentage of IMGs in the program:** 60%
**Minimum USMLE Step 1 Score Requirement:** 220
**Minimum USMLE Step 2 Score Requirement:** 220
**Attempts on any step:** No limits set
**CS required at time of application:** Yes including ECFMG certificate
**USCE Requirement:** Yes at least one month
**Cut-Off time since graduation:** 5 years
**Program offers couple match:** Yes
**Visas Sponsored or accepted:** J1 visa and H1b visa

## Beth Israel Deaconess Medical Center Internal Medicine Residency Program

**Specialty:** Internal Medicine
**Program name:** Beth Israel Deaconess Medical Center Program
**Program code:** 140-24-21-162
**NRMP Code:** 1256140C0, 1256140P0, 1256140P1, 1256140M0, 1256140M1
**Program type:** University-based
**State:** Massachusetts
**Address:** Beth Israel Deaconess Medical Center, 330 Brookline Ave, Boston, MA  02215
**Phone:** (617) 632-8273
**Fax:** (617) 632-8261

**Percentage of IMGs in the program:** 20%
**Minimum USMLE Step 1 Score Requirement:** 230
**Minimum USMLE Step 2 Score Requirement:** 230
**Attempts on any step:** Must pass on first attempt
**CS required at time of application:** Yes including ECFMG certificate
**USCE Requirement:** Yes, 1 year
**Cut-Off time since graduation:** 3 years
**Program offers couple match:** Yes
**Visas Sponsored or accepted:** J1 visa and H1b visa

## Tufts Medical Center Internal Medicine Residency Program

**Specialty:** Internal Medicine
**Program name:** Tufts Medical Center Program
**Program code:** 140-24-21-171
**NRMP Code:** 1263140C0
**Program type:** University-based
**State:** Massachusetts
**Address:** Tufts Med Center,
          800 Washington St, Boston, MA 02111
**Phone:** (617) 636-5246
**Fax:** (617) 636-7119
**Percentage of IMGs in the program:** 30%

**Minimum USMLE Step 1 Score Requirement:** 220
**Minimum USMLE Step 2 Score Requirement:** 220
**Attempts on any step:** Must pass on first attempt
**CS required at time of application:** Yes including ECFMG certificate
**USCE Requirement:** 3 months
**Cut-Off time since graduation:** 3 years
**Program offers couple match:** Yes
**Visas Sponsored or accepted:** J1 visa

## St Elizabeth's Medical Center Internal Medicine Residency Program

**Specialty:** Internal Medicine
**Program name:** St Elizabeth's Medical Center Program
**Program code:** 140-24-21-173
**State:** Massachusetts
**Address:** St Elizabeth's Medical Center,
        736 Cambridge St, Boston, MA  02135
**Phone:** (617) 562-7776
**Percentage of IMGs in the program:** 80%
**Minimum USMLE Step 1 Score Requirement:** 220
**Minimum USMLE Step 2 Score Requirement:**

**Attempts on any step:** No limits set
**CS required at time of application:** Yes
including ECFMG certificate
**USCE Requirement:** 1 month
**Cut-Off time since graduation:** 5 years
**Program offers couple match:** Yes
**Visas Sponsored or accepted:** J1 visa

## MetroWest Medical Center Internal Medicine Residency Program

**Specialty:** Internal Medicine
**Program name:** MetroWest Medical Center Program
**Program code:** 140-24-21-177
**NRMP Code:** 1812140C0
**Program type:** Community-based university affiliated hospital
**State:** Massachusetts
**Address:** MetroWest Medical Center
          115 Lincoln St, Framingham, MA 01702
**Phone:** (508) 383-1572
**Fax:** (508) 872-4794
**Percentage of IMGs in the program:** 100%
**Minimum USMLE Step 1 Score Requirement:** No limits set
**Minimum USMLE Step 2 Score Requirement:** No limits set

**Attempts on any step:** No limits set
**CS required at time of application:** No
**USCE Requirement:** 1-3 months with 3 US LORs
**Cut-Off time since graduation:** 5 years
**Program offers couple match:** Yes
**Visas Sponsored or accepted:** J1 visa

## University of Massachusetts Internal Medicine Residency Program

**Specialty:** Internal Medicine
**Program name:** University of Massachusetts Program
**Program code:** 140-24-21-184
**NRMP Code:** 3050140P1, 3050140P0, 3050140C0
**Program type:** University-based
**State:** Massachusetts
**Address:** University of Massachusetts Medical School
      55 Lake Ave N, Worcester, MA  01655
**Phone:** (774) 442-2173
**Fax:** (774) 442-6781
**Percentage of IMGs in the program:** 40%
**Minimum USMLE Step 1 Score Requirement:** No limits set
**Minimum USMLE Step 2 Score Requirement:** No limits set
**Attempts on any step:** Must pass on first

attempt
**CS required at time of application:** Yes
including ECFMG certificate
**USCE Requirement:** None
**Cut-Off time since graduation:** No limits set
**Program offers couple match:** Yes
**Visas Sponsored or accepted:** J1 visa

## Lahey Clinic Internal Medicine Residency Program

**Specialty:** Internal Medicine
**Program name:** Lahey Clinic Program
**Program code:** 140-24-21-511
**NRMP Code:** 3130140C0, 3130140P1, 3130140P0
**Program type:** Community-based university affiliated hospital
**State:** Massachusetts
**Address:** Lahey Hospital & Medical Center
41 Mall Rd, Burlington, MA  01805
**Phone:** (781) 744-5700
**Fax:** (781) 744-5358
**Percentage of IMGs in the program:** 40%
**Minimum USMLE Step 1 Score Requirement:** 210
**Minimum USMLE Step 2 Score Requirement:** 210
**Attempts on any step:** No limits set
**CS required at time of application:** No

**USCE Requirement:** Yes 1-3 months
**Cut-Off time since graduation:** No limits set
**Program offers couple match:** Yes
**Visas Sponsored or accepted:** J1 visa

## Boston Medical Center Internal Medicine Residency Program

**Specialty:** Internal Medicine
**Program name:** Boston Medical Center Program
**Program code:** 140-24-31-164
**NRMP Code:** 1257140P0, 1257140C0, 1257140M0
**Program type:** University-based
**State:** Massachusetts
**Address:** Boston University Medical Center
          72 E Concord St, Boston, MA  02118
**Phone:** (617) 638-6514
**Fax:** (617) 638-6501
**Percentage of IMGs in the program:** 10%
**Minimum USMLE Step 1 Score Requirement:** 210
**Minimum USMLE Step 2 Score Requirement:** 210
**Attempts on any step:** No limits set
**CS required at time of application:** Yes including ECFMG certificate
**USCE Requirement:** 2 months
**Cut-Off time since graduation:** 5 years

**Program offers couple match:** Yes
**Visas Sponsored or accepted:** J1 visa

# Michigan

## Wayne State University School of Medicine Internal Medicine Residency Program

**Specialty:** Internal Medicine
**Program name:** Wayne State University School of Medicine Program
**Program code:** 140-25-00-896
**NRMP Code:** 1361140C0
**Program type:** University-based
**State:** Michigan
**Address:** Crittenton Hospital Medical Center, 3 North GME Admin,
　　　1101 W University Dr, Rochester, MI 48307
**Phone:** (248) 601-4805
**Fax:** (248) 601-4908
**Percentage of IMGs in the program:** 80%
**Minimum USMLE Step 1 Score Requirement:** 220
**Minimum USMLE Step 2 Score Requirement:** 220
**Attempts on any step:** Must pass on first attempt including CS exam

**CS required at time of application:** No
**USCE Requirement:** None
**Cut-Off time since graduation:** 7 years
**Program offers couple match:** Yes
**Visas Sponsored or accepted:** J1 visa

## St. Mary Mercy Hospital Internal Medicine Residency Program

**Specialty:** Internal Medicine
**Program name:** St Mary Mercy Hospital Program
**Program code:** 140-25-12-540
**NRMP Code:** 1418140C0
**Program type:** Community-based
**State:** Michigan
**Address:** St Mary Mercy Hospital, GME Department,
  36475 Five Mile Rd, Livonia, MI  48154
**Phone:** (734) 655-2739
**Fax:** (734) 655-8430
**Percentage of IMGs in the program:** 70%
**Minimum USMLE Step 1 Score Requirement:** 200
**Minimum USMLE Step 2 Score Requirement:** 205
**Attempts on any step:** No limits set
**CS required at time of application:** No
**USCE Requirement:** None
**Cut-Off time since graduation:** 3 years

**Program offers couple match:** Yes
**Visas Sponsored or accepted:** J1 visa

## Providence Hospital and Medical Centers Internal Medicine Residency Program

**Specialty:** Internal Medicine
**Program name:** Providence Hospital and Medical Centers Program
**Program code:** 140-25-11-203
**NRMP Code:** 1303140C0
**Program type:** Community-based
**State:** Michigan
**Address:** Providence Hospital and Medical Center, PO Box 2043,
            16001 W Nine Mile Rd, Southfield, MI 48037
**Phone:** (248) 849-3151
**Fax:** (248) 849-3230
**Percentage of IMGs in the program:** 50%
**Minimum USMLE Step 1 Score Requirement:** 205
**Minimum USMLE Step 2 Score Requirement:** 205
**Attempts on any step:** Must pass on first attempt, but we do look at good CVs with attempts.
**CS required at time of application:** No

**USCE Requirement:** None
**Cut-Off time since graduation:** No limits set
**Program offers couple match:** No
**Visas Sponsored or accepted:** J1 visa and H1b visa

## Central Michigan University College of Medicine Internal Medicine Residency Program

**Specialty:** Internal Medicine
**Program name:** Central Michigan University College of Medicine Program
**Program code:** 140-25-31-202
**NRMP Code:** 1320140C0
**Program type:** University-based
**State:** Michigan
**Address:** Central Michigan University College of Medicine, Department of Internal Medicine, 1000 Houghton Ave, Saginaw, MI 48602
**Phone:** (989) 583-6826
**Fax:** (989) 583-6840
**Percentage of IMGs in the program:** 100%
**Minimum USMLE Step 1 Score Requirement:** 203
**Minimum USMLE Step 2 Score Requirement:** 204
**Attempts on any step:** No limits set
**CS required at time of application:** No

**USCE Requirement:** None
**Cut-Off time since graduation:** No limits set
**Program offers couple match:** No
**Visas Sponsored or accepted:** J1 visa

## William Beaumont Hospital Internal Medicine Residency Program

**Specialty:** Internal Medicine
**Program name:** William Beaumont Hospital Program
**Program code:** 140-25-12-201
**NRMP Code:** 1978140P0, 1978140C0
**Program type:** Community-based university affiliated hospital
**State:** Michigan
**Address:** William Beaumont Hospital, Department of Medicine,
          3601 W 13 Mile Rd, Royal Oak, MI 48073-6769
**Phone:** (248) 551-0406
**Fax:** (248) 551-8880
**Percentage of IMGs in the program:** 50%
**Minimum USMLE Step 1 Score Requirement:** No limits set
**Minimum USMLE Step 2 Score Requirement:** No limits set

**Attempts on any step:** Must pass on first attempt, but they look into good CVs with attempts.
**CS required at time of application:** No
**USCE Requirement:** None
**Cut-Off time since graduation:** No limits set
**Program offers couple match:** Yes
**Visas Sponsored or accepted:** J1 visa and H1b visa

## St. Joseph Mercy-Oakland Internal Medicine Residency Program

**Specialty:** Internal Medicine
**Program name:** St Joseph Mercy-Oakland Program
**Program code:** 140-25-11-200
**NRMP Code:** 1319140C0
**Program type:** Community-based university affiliated hospital
**State:** Michigan
**Address:** St Joseph Mercy Oakland, Department of Medicine,
          44405 Woodward Ave, Pontiac, MI 48341
**Phone:** (248) 858-6233
**Percentage of IMGs in the program:** 80%
**Minimum USMLE Step 1 Score Requirement:** 210

**Minimum USMLE Step 2 Score Requirement:** 210

**Attempts on any step:** Must pass on first attempt including CS exam

**CS required at time of application:** No

**USCE Requirement:** None

**Cut-Off time since graduation:** 5 years

**Program offers couple match:** Yes

**Visas Sponsored or accepted:** J1 visa

## Western Michigan University School of Medicine Internal Medicine Residency Program

**Specialty:** Internal Medicine

**Program name:** Western Michigan University School of Medicine Program

**Program code:** 140-25-21-199

**NRMP Code:** 1314140C0

**Program type:** Community-based university affiliated hospital

**State:** Michigan

**Address:** Western Michigan University School of Medicine, Internal Medicine Department, 1000 Oakland Dr, Kalamazoo, MI 49008

**Phone:** (269) 337-6361

**Fax:** (269) 337-6380

**Percentage of IMGs in the program:** 70%

**Minimum USMLE Step 1 Score Requirement:**
220
**Minimum USMLE Step 2 Score Requirement:**
220
**Attempts on any step:** Must pass on first
attempt
**CS required at time of application:** No
**USCE Requirement:** None
**Cut-Off time since graduation:** 5 years unless in
residency or clinically active
**Program offers couple match:** Yes
**Visas Sponsored or accepted:** J1 visa and H1b
visa

## Grand Rapids Medical Education Partners/Michigan State University Internal Medicine Residency Program

**Specialty:** Internal Medicine
**Program name:** Grand Rapids Medical
Education Partners/Michigan State University
Program
**Program code:** 140-25-31-198
**NRMP Code:** 2077140C0
**Program type:** Community-based university
affiliated hospital
**State:** Michigan
**Address:** Grand Rapids Medical Education
Partners, Suite 2200,

25 Michigan Ave NE, Grand Rapids, MI  49503
**Phone:** (616) 391-3246
**Percentage of IMGs in the program:** 75%
**Minimum USMLE Step 1 Score Requirement:** 206
**Minimum USMLE Step 2 Score Requirement:** 206
**Attempts on any step:** No limits set
**CS required at time of application:** No
**USCE Requirement:** None
**Cut-Off time since graduation:** 3 years unless in residency or clinically active
**Program offers couple match:** Yes
**Visas Sponsored or accepted:** J1 visa

## McLaren Regional Medical Center/Michigan State University Internal Medicine Residency Program

**Specialty:** Internal Medicine
**Program name:** McLaren-Flint/Michigan State University Program
**Program code:** 140-25-21-471
**Program type:** Community-based university affiliated hospital
**State:** Michigan
**Address:** McLaren Regional Medical Center, Department of Medicine,
401 S Ballenger Hwy, Flint, MI  48532
**Phone:** (810) 342-2968

**Fax:** (810) 342-4976
**Percentage of IMGs in the program:** 100%
**Minimum USMLE Step 1 Score Requirement:** 205
**Minimum USMLE Step 2 Score Requirement:** 205
**Attempts on any step:** Allow only one failed attempt total on Step 1 and 2 CK combined.
**CS required at time of application:** No
**USCE Requirement:** No
**Cut-Off time since graduation:** 7 years
**Program offers couple match:** Yes
**Visas Sponsored or accepted:** J1 visa

## Hurley Medical Center/Michigan State University Internal Medicine Residency Program

**Specialty:** Internal Medicine
**Program name:** Hurley Medical Center/Michigan State University Program
**Program code:** 140-25-31-196
**NRMP Code:** 1307140C0
**Program type:** Community-based university affiliated hospital
**State:** Michigan
**Address:** Hurley Medical Center, Suite 212, Two Hurley Plaza, Flint, MI  48503
**Phone:** (810) 262-9080
**Fax:** (810) 262-7245

**Percentage of IMGs in the program:** 60%
**Minimum USMLE Step 1 Score Requirement:** 213
**Minimum USMLE Step 2 Score Requirement:** 212
**Attempts on any step:** Must pass on first attempt, but they accept good profiles with attempts.
**CS required at time of application:** Yes
**USCE Requirement:** None
**Cut-Off time since graduation:** 5 years
**Program offers couple match:** Yes
**Visas Sponsored or accepted:** J1 visa and H1b visa

## Michigan State University Internal Medicine Residency Program

**Specialty:** Internal Medicine
**Program name:** Michigan State University Program
**Program code:** 140-25-21-195
**NRMP Code:** 2436140C0
**Program type:** Community-based university affiliated hospital
**State:** Michigan
**Address:** Michigan State University, Clinical Center Room B301,
788 Service Rd, East Lansing, MI 48824

**Phone:** (517) 353-5100
**Fax:** (517) 432-2759
**Percentage of IMGs in the program:** 60%
**Minimum USMLE Step 1 Score Requirement:** No limits set
**Minimum USMLE Step 2 Score Requirement:** No limits set
**Attempts on any step:** No limits set
**CS required at time of application:** Yes including ECFMG certificate
**USCE Requirement:** None
**Cut-Off time since graduation:** 2 years unless in residency or clinically active
**Program offers couple match:** Yes
**Visas Sponsored or accepted:** J1 visa

## Detroit Medical Center/Wayne State University Internal Medicine Residency Program

**Specialty:** Internal Medicine
**Program name:** Detroit Medical Center/Wayne State University Program
**Program code:** 140-25-21-194
**NRMP Code:** 1295140C0
**Program type:** University-based
**State:** Michigan
**Address:** Detroit Med Center/Wayne State University, UHC Suite 2E,

4201 St Antoine Blvd, Detroit, MI 48201
**Phone:** (313) 745-7999
**Fax:** (313) 745-4052
**Percentage of IMGs in the program:** 65%
**Minimum USMLE Step 1 Score Requirement:** No limits set
**Minimum USMLE Step 2 Score Requirement:** No limits set
**Attempts on any step:** Must pass on first attempt
**CS required at time of application:** Yes including ECFMG certificate
**USCE Requirement:** 2 months
**Cut-Off time since graduation:** 3 years unless in residency
**Program offers couple match:** Yes
**Visas Sponsored or accepted:** J1 visa

## St. John Hospital and Medical Center Internal Medicine Residency Program

**Specialty:** Internal Medicine
**Program name:** St John Hospital and Medical Center Program
**Program code:** 140-25-11-191
**NRMP Code:** 1915140C0, 1915140P0
**Program type:** Community-based university affiliated hospital

**State:** Michigan
**Address:** St John Hospital and Medical Center,
Department of Medicine Education,
Suite 340,
19251 Mack Ave, Grosse Pointe
Woods, MI  48236
**Phone:** (313) 343-3875
**Fax:** (313) 343-7840
**Percentage of IMGs in the program:** 40%
**Minimum USMLE Step 1 Score Requirement:**
No limits set
**Minimum USMLE Step 2 Score Requirement:**
No limits set
**Attempts on any step:** Must pass on first
attempt including CS exam
**CS required at time of application:** No
**USCE Requirement:** None
**Cut-Off time since graduation:** 5 years unless in
residency or clinically active
**Program offers couple match:** Yes
**Visas Sponsored or accepted:** J1 visa and H1b
visa

## Henry Ford Hospital/Wayne State University Internal Medicine Residency Program

**Specialty:** Internal Medicine
**Program name:** Henry Ford Hospital/Wayne
State University Program

**Program code:** 140-25-11-189
**State:** Michigan
**Address:** Henry Ford Hospital, Department of Medicine CFP-1,
2799 W Grand Blvd, Detroit, MI 48202
**Phone:** (313) 916-1888
**Fax:** (313) 916-1394
**Percentage of IMGs in the program:** 70%
**Minimum USMLE Step 1 Score Requirement:** No limits set
**Minimum USMLE Step 2 Score Requirement:** No limits set
**Attempts on any step:** Must pass first attempt
**CS required at time of application:** No
**USCE Requirement:** None
**Cut-Off time since graduation:** 4 years
**Program offers couple match:** Yes
**Visas Sponsored or accepted:** J1 visa

## Detroit Medical Center/Wayne State University (Sinai-Grace) Internal Medicine Residency Program

**Specialty:** Internal Medicine
**Program name:** Detroit Medical Center/Wayne State University (Sinai-Grace) Program
**Program code:** 140-25-21-506
**NRMP Code:** 1374140C0

**Program type:** Community-based university affiliated hospital
**State:** Michigan
**Address:** Sinai-Grace Hospital, Department of Medicine,
6071 W Outer Dr, Detroit, MI 48235
**Phone:** (313) 966-7434
**Fax:** (313) 966-1738
**Percentage of IMGs in the program:** 50%
**Minimum USMLE Step 1 Score Requirement:** 205
**Minimum USMLE Step 2 Score Requirement:** 205
**Attempts on any step:** Must pass on first attempt
**CS required at time of application:** No
**USCE Requirement:** No
**Cut-Off time since graduation:** 4 years unless in residency or clinically active
**Program offers couple match:** Yes
**Visas Sponsored or accepted:** J1 visa

## Oakwood Hospital Internal Medicine Residency Program

**Specialty:** Internal Medicine
**Program name:** Oakwood Hospital Program
**Program code:** 140-25-31-188
**NRMP Code:** 1946140C0, 1946140P0
**Program type:** Community-based

**State:** Michigan
**Address:** Oakwood Hospital and Medical Center, Internal Medicine Program,
 18101 Oakwood Blvd, Dearborn, MI 48124
**Phone:** (313) 436-2578
**Fax:** (313) 436-2071
**Percentage of IMGs in the program:** 50%
**Minimum USMLE Step 1 Score Requirement:** 210
**Minimum USMLE Step 2 Score Requirement:** 210
**Attempts on any step:** Must pass on first attempt including CS exam
**CS required at time of application:** Yes
**USCE Requirement:** Yes
**Cut-Off time since graduation:** 5 years
**Program offers couple match:** Yes
**Visas Sponsored or accepted:** No

## St. Joseph Mercy Hospital Internal Medicine Residency Program

**Specialty:** Internal Medicine
**Program name:** St Joseph Mercy Hospital Program
**Program code:** 140-25-12-186
**NRMP Code:** 1292140C0, 1292140P0

**Program type:** Community-based university affiliated hospital
**State:** Michigan
**Address:** St Joseph Mercy Hospital, PO Box 995, 5333 McAuley Dr, Ann Arbor, MI 48106
**Phone:** (734) 712-3935
**Fax:** (734) 712-5583
**Percentage of IMGs in the program:** 80%
**Minimum USMLE Step 1 Score Requirement:** 210
**Minimum USMLE Step 2 Score Requirement:** 210
**Attempts on any step:** Must pass on first attempt including CS exam
**CS required at time of application:** No
**USCE Requirement:** None
**Cut-Off time since graduation:** 3 years
**Program offers couple match:** Yes
**Visas Sponsored or accepted:** J1 visa

## Minnesota

### University of Minnesota Internal Medicine Residency Program

**Specialty:** Internal Medicine
**Program name:** University of Minnesota Program
**Program code:** 140-26-21-205
**NRMP Code:** 1334140C0
**Program type:** University-based
**State:** Minnesota
**Address:** University of Minnesota Medical Center,

    420 Delaware St SE, Minneapolis, MN 55455
**Phone:** (612) 625-5454
**Fax:** (612) 625-3238
**Percentage of IMGs in the program:** 20%
**Minimum USMLE Step 1 Score Requirement:** No limits set
**Minimum USMLE Step 2 Score Requirement:** No limits set
**Attempts on any step:** Must pass on first attempt
**CS required at time of application:** Yes including ECFMG certificate
**USCE Requirement:** None
**Cut-Off time since graduation:** No limits set
**Program offers couple match:** Yes
**Visas Sponsored or accepted:** J1 visa

# Abbott-Northwestern Hospital Internal Medicine Residency Program

**Specialty:** Internal Medicine
**Program name:** Abbott-Northwestern Hospital Program
**Program code:** 140-26-31-204
**NRMP Code:** 1330140C0
**Program type:** Community-based university affiliated hospital
**State:** Minnesota
**Address:** Abbott-Northwestern Hospital
800 E 28th St, Minneapolis, MN 55407-3799
**Phone:** (612) 863-6766
**Percentage of IMGs in the program:** 10%
**Minimum USMLE Step 1 Score Requirement:** 220
**Minimum USMLE Step 2 Score Requirement:** 220
**Attempts on any step:** Must pass on first attempt including CS exam
**CS required at time of application:** Yes including ECFMG certificate
**USCE Requirement:** None
**Cut-Off time since graduation:** 1 year
**Program offers couple match:** Yes
**Visas Sponsored or accepted:** J1 visa

# Hennepin County Medical Center Internal Medicine Residency Program

**Specialty:** Internal Medicine
**Program name:** Hennepin County Medical Center Program
**Program code:** 140-26-31-207
**NRMP Code:** 1329140C0
**Program type:** Community-based university affiliated hospital
**State:** Minnesota
**Address:** Hennepin County Medical Center
         701 Park Ave S, Minneapolis, MN 55415
**Phone:** (612) 873-4733
**Fax:** (612) 904-4577
**Percentage of IMGs in the program:** 20%
**Minimum USMLE Step 1 Score Requirement:** 210
**Minimum USMLE Step 2 Score Requirement:** 210
**Attempts on any step:** Must pass on first attempt
**CS required at time of application:** Yes including ECFMG certificate
**USCE Requirement:** Yes 8 weeks
**Cut-Off time since graduation:** 5 years
**Program offers couple match:** Yes
**Visas Sponsored or accepted:** J1 visa

# Mississippi

## University of Mississippi Medical Center Internal Medicine Residency Program

**Specialty:** Internal Medicine
**Program name:** University of Mississippi Medical Center Program
**Program code:** 140-27-21-209
**NRMP Code:** 1957140P2, 1957140C0, 1957140M0, 1957140P0
**Program type:** University-based
**State:** Mississippi
**Address:** University of Mississippi Medical Center
           2500 N State St, Jackson, MS 39216-4505
**Phone:** (601) 984-5601
**Fax:** (601) 984-6665
**Percentage of IMGs in the program:** 20%
**Minimum USMLE Step 1 Score Requirement:** No limits set
**Minimum USMLE Step 2 Score Requirement:** No limits set
**Attempts on any step:** No limits set

**CS required at time of application:** Yes including ECFMG certificate
**USCE Requirement:** None
**Cut-Off time since graduation:** 5 years
**Program offers couple match:** Yes
**Visas Sponsored or accepted:** J1 visa

## Missouri

### St Mary's Health Center Internal Medicine Residency Program

**Specialty:** Internal Medicine
**Program name:** St Mary's Health Center Program
**Program code:** 140-28-11-220
**NRMP Code:** 1999140P0, 1999140C0
**Program type:** Community-based university affiliated hospital
**State:** Missouri
**Address:** St Mary's Health Center,
　　　　6420 Clayton Rd, St Louis, MO  63117
**Phone:** (314) 768-8778
**Fax:** (314) 768-7101
**Percentage of IMGs in the program:** 70%
**Minimum USMLE Step 1 Score Requirement:** 210
**Minimum USMLE Step 2 Score Requirement:**

**Attempts on any step:** Must pass n first attempt
**CS required at time of application:** Yes including ECFMG certificate
**USCE Requirement:** None
**Cut-Off time since graduation:** 7 years
**Program offers couple match:** Yes
**Visas Sponsored or accepted:** J1 visa and H1b visa

## University of Missouri-Columbia Internal Medicine Residency Program

**Specialty:** Internal Medicine
**Program name:** University of Missouri-Columbia Program
**Program code:** 140-28-21-210
**NRMP Code:** 1994140C0, 1994140P0
**Program type:** University-based
**State:** Missouri
**Address:** University of Missouri-Columbia
            One Hospital Dr, Columbia, MO  65212
**Phone:** (573) 884-1606
**Fax:** (573) 884-5690
**Percentage of IMGs in the program:** 25%
**Minimum USMLE Step 1 Score Requirement:** 225
**Minimum USMLE Step 2 Score Requirement:**

**Attempts on any step:** Must pass on first attempt
**CS required at time of application:** Yes including ECFMG certificate
**USCE Requirement:** None
**Cut-Off time since graduation:** 5 years
**Program offers couple match:** Yes
**Visas Sponsored or accepted:** J1 visa (and H1b visa for outstanding applicants)

# St Louis University School of Medicine Internal Medicine Residency Program

**Specialty:** Internal Medicine
**Program name:** St Louis University School of Medicine Program
**Program code:** 140-28-21-218
**NRMP Code:** 1365140P0, 1365140C0
**Program type:** University-based
**State:** Missouri
**Address:** St Louis University School of Medicine 1402 S Grand Blvd, St Louis, MO 63104
**Phone:** (314) 577-8762
**Fax:** (314) 577-8100
**Percentage of IMGs in the program:** 0% (Varies from 0-30%)

**Minimum USMLE Step 1 Score Requirement:** 213

**Minimum USMLE Step 2 Score Requirement:** 213

**Attempts on any step:** Must pass on the first attempt

**CS required at time of application:** No

**USCE Requirement:** Yes at least 1 month within the last year

**Cut-Off time since graduation:** 5 years

**Program offers couple match:** Yes

**Visas Sponsored or accepted:** J1 visa (and H1b visa for select candidates)

## St Luke's Hospital Internal Medicine Residency Program

**Specialty:** Internal Medicine

**Program name:** St Luke's Hospital Internal Medicine Residency Program

**Program code:** 140-28-21-219

**NRMP Code:** 1364140P0, 1364140C0

**Program type:** Community-based university affiliated hospital

**State:** Missouri

**Address:** St Luke's Hospital
          222 S Woods Mill Rd, St Louis, MO 63017

**Phone:** (314) 205-6050

**Fax:** (314) 434-5939

**Percentage of IMGs in the program:** 95%
**Minimum USMLE Step 1 Score Requirement:** 210
**Minimum USMLE Step 2 Score Requirement:** 210
**Attempts on any step:** Must pass on the first attempt
**CS required at time of application:** Yes including ECFMG certificate
**USCE Requirement:** None
**Cut-Off time since graduation:** 5 years
**Program offers couple match:** Yes
**Visas Sponsored or accepted:** J1 visa and H1b visa

## University of Missouri at Kansas City Internal Medicine Residency Program

**Specialty:** Internal Medicine
**Program name:** University of Missouri at Kansas City Program
**Program code:** 140-28-31-214
**NRMP Code:** 1343140C0, 1343140P0
**Program type:** University-based
**State:** Missouri
**Address:** UMKC School of Medicine,
          2411 Holmes St, Kansas City, MO 64108
**Phone:** (816) 932-3406

**Fax:** (816) 932-5179
**Percentage of IMGs in the program:** 80%
**Minimum USMLE Step 1 Score Requirement:** 225
**Minimum USMLE Step 2 Score Requirement:** 225
**Attempts on any step:** Must pass on the first attempt
**CS required at time of application:** Yes including ECFMG certificate
**USCE Requirement:** At least 1 month in the last 1 year
**Cut-Off time since graduation:** 5 years
**Program offers couple match:** Yes
**Visas Sponsored or accepted:** J1 visa

## Mercy Hospital (St Louis) Internal Medicine Residency Program

**Specialty:** Internal Medicine
**Program name:** Mercy Hospital (St Louis) Program
**Program code:** 140-28-31-217
**NRMP Code:** 1362140C0
**Program type:** Community-based university affiliated hospital
**State:** Missouri
**Address:** Mercy Hospital St Louis
          621 S New Ballas Rd, St Louis, MO 63141-8277

**Phone:** (314) 251-5834
**Fax:** (314) 251-6272
**Percentage of IMGs in the program:** 20%
**Minimum USMLE Step 1 Score Requirement:** 220
**Minimum USMLE Step 2 Score Requirement:** 220
**Attempts on any step:** No limits set
**CS required at time of application:** Yes including ECFMG certificate
**USCE Requirement:** Yes 6 months with at least 1 US LOR
**Cut-Off time since graduation:** 5 years
**Program offers couple match:** Yes
**Visas Sponsored or accepted:** H1b visa


# Montana


## Billings Clinic Internal Medicine Residency Program

**Specialty:** Internal Medicine
**Program name:** Billings Clinic Program
**Program code:** 140-29-00-919
**NRMP Code:** 1633140C0, 1633140P0
**Program type:** Community-based
**State:** Montana
**Address:** Billings Clinic
        2800 Tenth Ave N, Billings, MT  59107-

7000
**Phone:** (406) 238-2210
**Fax:** (406) 238-5832
**Percentage of IMGs in the program:** 30%
**Minimum USMLE Step 1 Score Requirement:**
No limits set
**Minimum USMLE Step 2 Score Requirement:**
No limits set
**Attempts on any step:** No limits set
**CS required at time of application:** No
**USCE Requirement:** None
**Cut-Off time since graduation:** No limits set
**Program offers couple match:** Yes
**Visas Sponsored or accepted:** J1 visa

# Nebraska

## Creighton University Internal Medicine Residency Program

**Specialty:** Internal Medicine
**Program name:** Creighton University Program
**Program code:** 140-30-21-222
**NRMP Code:** 1372140P0, 1372140C0

**Program type:** University-based
**State:** Nebraska
**Address:** Alegent Creighton University Medical Center
        601 N 30th St, Omaha, NE  68131-2197
**Phone:** (402) 280-4210
**Percentage of IMGs in the program:** 70%
**Minimum USMLE Step 1 Score Requirement:** No limits set
**Minimum USMLE Step 2 Score Requirement:** No limits set
**Attempts on any step:** Must pass on first attempt
**CS required at time of application:** Yes including ECFMG certificate
**USCE Requirement:** None but preferred
**Cut-Off time since graduation:** 5 years
**Program offers couple match:** Yes
**Visas Sponsored or accepted:** J1 visa

## University of Nebraska Medical Center College of Medicine Internal Medicine Residency Program

**Specialty:** Internal Medicine
**Program name:** University of Nebraska Medical Center College of Medicine Program
**Program code:** 140-30-21-224
**NRMP Code:** 1376140C0, 1376140P0
**Program type:** University-based

**State:** Nebraska
**Address:** University of Nebraska Medical Center
982055 Nebraska Medical Center,
Omaha, NE  68198-2055
**Phone:** (402) 559-7268
**Fax:** (402) 559-9385
**Percentage of IMGs in the program:** 20%
**Minimum USMLE Step 1 Score Requirement:**
No limits set
**Minimum USMLE Step 2 Score Requirement:**
No limits set
**Attempts on any step:** No limits set
**CS required at time of application:** Yes
including ECFMG certificate
**USCE Requirement:** None
**Cut-Off time since graduation:** No limits set
**Program offers couple match:** Yes
**Visas Sponsored or accepted:** J1 visa and H1b
visa

# Nevada

# University of Nevada School of Medicine Internal Medicine Residency Program

**Specialty:** Internal Medicine
**Program name:** University of Nevada School of Medicine Program
**Program code:** 140-31-21-483
**NRMP Code:** 2017140C0, 2017140P0
**Program type:** Community-based university affiliated hospital
**State:** Nevada
**Address:** University of Nevada Reno
            1155 Mill St, Reno, NV  89502
**Phone**: (775) 327-5174
**Fax:** (775) 327-5178
**Percentage of IMGs in the program:** 40%
**Minimum USMLE Step 1 Score Requirement:** 200
**Minimum USMLE Step 2 Score Requirement:** 210
**Attempts on any step:** Must pass on the first attempt
**CS required at time of application:** Yes including ECFMG certificate
**USCE Requirement:** 6 weeks
**Cut-Off time since graduation:** 5 years but not strict
**Program offers couple match:** Yes
**Visas Sponsored or accepted:** No visa

# University of Nevada School of Medicine (Las Vegas) Internal Medicine Residency Program

**Specialty:** Internal Medicine
**Program name:** University of Nevada School of Medicine (Las Vegas) Program
**Program code:** 140-31-21-497
**NRMP Code:** 2028140P0, 2028140C0
**Program type:** Community-based university affiliated hospital
**State:** Nevada
**Address:** University of Nevada School of Medicine

       2040 W Charleston Blvd, Las Vegas, NV 89102
**Phone:** (702) 671-2345
**Fax:** (702) 671-2376
**Percentage of IMGs in the program:** 80%
**Minimum USMLE Step 1 Score Requirement:** 205
**Minimum USMLE Step 2 Score Requirement:** 205
**Attempts on any step:** Must pass maximum on 3rd attempt on any step
**CS required at time of application:** Yes including ECFMG certificate
**USCE Requirement:** None
**Cut-Off time since graduation:** 5 years, but if clinically active in the past 5 years then 8 years
**Program offers couple match:** Yes

**Visas Sponsored or accepted:** J1 visa and H1b visa

# New Jersey

## Monmouth Medical Center Internal Medicine Residency Program

**Specialty:** Internal Medicine
**Program name:** Monmouth Medical Center Program
**Program code:** 140-33-11-233
**NRMP Code:** 1392140C0
**Program type:** Community-based university affiliated hospital
**State:** New Jersey
**Address:** Monmouth Medical Center,
        300 Second Ave, Long Branch, NJ 07740-9998
**Phone:** (732) 923-6537
**Fax:** (732) 923-6536
**Percentage of IMGs in the program:** 90%
**Minimum USMLE Step 1 Score Requirement:** 210
**Minimum USMLE Step 2 Score Requirement:** 210
**Attempts on any step:** No limits set

**CS required at time of application:** Yes
**USCE Requirement:** None
**Cut-Off time since graduation:** No limits set
**Program offers couple match:** Yes
**Visas Sponsored or accepted:** J1 visa

## HackensackUMC Mountainside Internal Medicine Residency Program

**Specialty:** Internal Medicine
**Program name:** HackensackUMC Mountainside Program
**Program code:** 140-33-11-234
**NRMP Code:** 1393140C0
**Program type:** Community-based university affiliated hospital
**State:** New Jersey
**Address:** HackensackUMC Mountainside
One Bay Ave, Montclair, NJ  07042
**Phone:** (973) 680-7860
**Fax:** (973) 429-6575
**Percentage of IMGs in the program:** 100%
**Minimum USMLE Step 1 Score Requirement:** 210
**Minimum USMLE Step 2 Score Requirement:** 210
**Attempts on any step:** Must pass on first attempt
**CS required at time of application:** Yes

including ECFMG certificate
**USCE Requirement:** None
**Cut-Off time since graduation:** 5 years
**Program offers couple match:** Yes
**Visas Sponsored or accepted:** No visa

## Atlantic Health (Morristown) Internal Medicine Residency Program

**Specialty:** Internal Medicine
**Program name:** Atlantic Health (Morristown)
Program
**Program code:** 140-33-11-235
**NRMP Code:** 1394140C0, 1394140P0
**Program type:** Community-based university
affiliated hospital
**State:** New Jersey
**Address:** Morristown Medical Center,
          100 Madison Ave, Morristown, NJ
07962-1956
**Phone:** (973) 971-4102
**Fax:** (973) 290-8325
**Percentage of IMGs in the program:** 70%
**Minimum USMLE Step 1 Score Requirement:**
No limits set
**Minimum USMLE Step 2 Score Requirement:**
No limits set
**Attempts on any step:** No limits set
**CS required at time of application:** Yes

including ECFMG certificate
**USCE Requirement:** None
**Cut-Off time since graduation:** 5 years unless clinically active
**Program offers couple match:** Yes
**Visas Sponsored or accepted:** J1 visa


## Atlantic Health (Overlook) Internal Medicine Residency Program

**Specialty:** Internal Medicine
**Program name:** Atlantic Health (Overlook) Program
**Program code:** 140-33-11-245
**NRMP Code:** 1408140C0, 1408140P0
**Program type:** Community-based university affiliated hospital
**State:** New Jersey
**Address:** Overlook Medical Center
99 Beauvoir Ave, Summit, NJ 07902-0220
**Phone:** (908) 522-2987
**Fax:** (908) 522-0804
**Percentage of IMGs in the program:** 70%
**Minimum USMLE Step 1 Score Requirement:** No limits set
**Minimum USMLE Step 2 Score Requirement:** No limits set
**Attempts on any step:** No limits set
**CS required at time of application:** No

**USCE Requirement:** None
**Cut-Off time since graduation:** No limits set
**Program offers couple match:** Yes
**Visas Sponsored or accepted:** J1 visa and H1b visa

## Jersey Shore University Medical Center Internal Medicine Residency Program

**Specialty:** Internal Medicine
**Program name:** Jersey Shore University Medical Center Program
**Program code:** 140-33-12-236
**NRMP Code:** 1395140C0, 1395140P0
**Program type:** Community-based university affiliated hospital
**State:** New Jersey
**Address:** Jersey Shore University Medical Center
         1945 State Rte 33, Neptune, NJ  07754
**Phone:** (732) 776-4483
**Fax:** (732) 776-4798
**Percentage of IMGs in the program:** 70%
**Minimum USMLE Step 1 Score Requirement:** 225
**Minimum USMLE Step 2 Score Requirement:** 225
**Attempts on any step:** Must pass on first attempt

**CS required at time of application:** No
**USCE Requirement:** None
**Cut-Off time since graduation:** 10 years
**Program offers couple match:** Yes
**Visas Sponsored or accepted:** No visa

## St Barnabas Medical Center Internal Medicine Residency Program

**Specialty:** Internal Medicine
**Program name:** St Barnabas Medical Center Program
**Program code:** 140-33-12-457
**State:** New Jersey
**Address:** St Barnabas Medical Center
94 Old Short Hills Rd, Livingston, NJ 07039
**Phone:** (973) 322-5645
**Fax:** (973) 322-8215
**Percentage of IMGs in the program:** 90%
**Minimum USMLE Step 1 Score Requirement:** No limits set
**Minimum USMLE Step 2 Score Requirement:** No limits set
**Attempts on any step:** No limits set
**CS required at time of application:** Yes including ECFMG certificate
**USCE Requirement:** None
**Cut-Off time since graduation:** No limits set
**Program offers couple match:** Yes

**Visas Sponsored or accepted:** No visa ( J1 visa for outstanding applicants)

## Seton Hall University School of Health and Medical Sciences (St Francis) Internal Medicine Residency Program

**Specialty:** Internal Medicine
**Program name:** Seton Hall University School of Health and Medical Sciences (St Francis) Program
**Program code:** 140-33-13-523
**NRMP Code:** 3194140C1
**Program type:** Community-based
**State:** New Jersey
**Address:** St Francis Medical Center,
        601 Hamilton Ave, Trenton, NJ  08629-1986
**Phone:** (609) 599-5061
**Fax:** (609) 599-6232
**Percentage of IMGs in the program:** 80%
**Minimum USMLE Step 1 Score Requirement:** 220
**Minimum USMLE Step 2 Score Requirement:** 220
**Attempts on any step:** No limits set
**CS required at time of application:** No
**USCE Requirement:** None
**Cut-Off time since graduation:** No limits set

**Program offers couple match:** Yes
**Visas Sponsored or accepted:** J1 visa

## Cooper Medical School of Rowan University/Cooper University Hospital Internal Medicine Residency Program

**Specialty:** Internal Medicine
**Program name:** Cooper Medical School of Rowan University/Cooper University Hospital Program
**Program code:** 140-33-21-227
**NRMP Code:** 1380140M0, 1380140P0, 1380140C0
**Program type:** University-based
**State:** New Jersey
**Address:** Cooper University Hospital,
         401 Haddon Ave, Camden, NJ  08103
**Phone:** (856) 757-7842
**Fax:** (856) 968-9587
**Percentage of IMGs in the program:** 50%
**Minimum USMLE Step 1 Score Requirement:** 205
**Minimum USMLE Step 2 Score Requirement:** 205
**Attempts on any step:** No limits set
**CS required at time of application:** No
**USCE Requirement:** 6 months given preference
**Cut-Off time since graduation:** 5 years given

preference
**Program offers couple match:** Yes
**Visas Sponsored or accepted:** J1 visa

## Icahn School of Medicine at Mount Sinai (Englewood) Internal Medicine Residency Program

**Specialty:** Internal Medicine
**Program name:** Icahn School of Medicine at Mount Sinai (Englewood) Program
**Program code:** 140-33-21-228
**NRMP Code:** 1386140C0, 1386140P0
**Program type:** Community-based university affiliated hospital
**State:** New Jersey
**Address:** Englewood Hospital and Medical Center

350 Engle St, Englewood, NJ  07631-5479
**Phone:** (201) 894-3664
**Fax:** (201) 894-0839
**Percentage of IMGs in the program:** 90%
**Minimum USMLE Step 1 Score Requirement:** 205
**Minimum USMLE Step 2 Score Requirement:** 205
**Attempts on any step:** Must pass on first attempt
**CS required at time of application:** No

**USCE Requirement:** None
**Cut-Off time since graduation:** 7 years
**Program offers couple match:** Yes
**Visas Sponsored or accepted:** J1 visa

## Newark Beth Israel Medical Center (Jersey City) Internal Medicine Residency Program

**Specialty:** Internal Medicine
**Program name:** Newark Beth Israel Medical Center (Jersey City) Program
**Program code:** 140-33-21-232
**State:** New Jersey
**Address:** Jersey City Medical Center,
            355 Grand St, Jersey City, NJ  07302
**Phone:** (201) 915-2431
**Fax:** (201) 915-2219
**Percentage of IMGs in the program:** 90%
**Minimum USMLE Step 1 Score Requirement:** 212 but not strict
**Minimum USMLE Step 2 Score Requirement:** 212 but not strict
**Attempts on any step:** No limits set but prefer passing on first attempt
**CS required at time of application:** No
**USCE Requirement:** None
**Cut-Off time since graduation:** 3 years
**Program offers couple match:** Yes
**Visas Sponsored or accepted:** H1b visa

# Rutgers New Jersey Medical School Internal Medicine Residency Program

**Specialty:** Internal Medicine
**Program name:** Rutgers New Jersey Medical School Program
**Program code:** 140-33-21-237
**NRMP Code:** 1398140C0, 1398140P0, 1398140P2
**Program type:** University-based
**State:** New Jersey
**Address:** Rutgers New Jersey Medical School
             150 Bergen St, Newark, NJ  07103
**Phone:** (973) 972-2449
**Fax:** (973) 972-3129
**Percentage of IMGs in the program:** 20%
**Minimum USMLE Step 1 Score Requirement:** No limits set
**Minimum USMLE Step 2 Score Requirement:** No limits set
**Attempts on any step:** No limits set
**CS required at time of application:** No
**USCE Requirement:** None
**Cut-Off time since graduation:** No limits set but 3 years preferred
**Program offers couple match:** Yes
**Visas Sponsored or accepted:** J1 visa

# Rutgers Robert Wood Johnson Medical School Internal Medicine Residency Program

**Specialty:** Internal Medicine
**Program name:** Rutgers Robert Wood Johnson Medical School Program
**Program code:** 140-33-21-243
**NRMP Code:** 2918140C0, 2918140P0
**Program type:** University-based
**State:** New Jersey
**Address:** Rutgers Robert Wood Johnson Medical School
        One Robert Wood Johnson Pl, New Brunswick, NJ  08903-0019
**Phone:** (732) 235-7742
**Fax:**  (732) 235-7427
**Percentage of IMGs in the program:** 40%
**Minimum USMLE Step 1 Score Requirement:** 210
**Minimum USMLE Step 2 Score Requirement:** 210
**Attempts on any step:** Must pass on first attempt
**CS required at time of application:** No
**USCE Requirement:** None
**Cut-Off time since graduation:** 5 years
**Program offers couple match:** Yes
**Visas Sponsored or accepted:** J1 visa

# Capital Health Regional Medical Center Internal Medicine Residency Program

**Specialty:** Internal Medicine
**Program name:** Capital Health Regional Medical Center Program
**Program code:** 140-33-21-246
**NRMP Code:** 2003140C0
**Program type:** Community-based
**State:** New Jersey
**Address:** Capital Health Regional Medical Center,
            750 Brunswick Ave, Trenton, NJ 08638
**Phone:** (609) 394-6031
**Fax:** (609) 394-6028
**Percentage of IMGs in the program:** 100%
**Minimum USMLE Step 1 Score Requirement:** 205
**Minimum USMLE Step 2 Score Requirement:** 205
**Attempts on any step:** Must pass on first attempt
**CS required at time of application:** Yes including ECFMG certificate
**USCE Requirement:** None
**Cut-Off time since graduation:** No limits set but preferred 10 years
**Program offers couple match:** Yes
**Visas Sponsored or accepted:** No visa

## Raritan Bay Medical Center Internal Medicine Residency Program

**Specialty:** Internal Medicine
**Program name:** Raritan Bay Medical Center Program
**Program code:** 140-33-21-466
**NRMP Code:** 1873140C0
**Program type:** Community-based university affiliated hospital
**State:** New Jersey
**Address:** Raritan Bay Medical Center-Perth Amboy Division

       530 New Brunswick Ave, Perth Amboy, NJ  08861-3685
**Phone:** (732) 324-5080
**Fax:** (732) 324-4669
**Percentage of IMGs in the program:** 100%
**Minimum USMLE Step 1 Score Requirement:** No limits set
**Minimum USMLE Step 2 Score Requirement:** No limits set
**Attempts on any step:** No limits set
**CS required at time of application:** Yes including ECFMG certificate
**USCE Requirement:** None
**Cut-Off time since graduation:** No limits set
**Program offers couple match:** No
**Visas Sponsored or accepted:** No visa

# Seton Hall University School of Health and Medical Sciences Internal Medicine Residency Program

**Specialty:** Internal Medicine
**Program name:** Seton Hall University School of Health and Medical Sciences Program
**Program code:** 140-33-21-498
**NRMP Code:** 3194140C0, 3194140C2
**Program type:** Community-based
**State:** New Jersey
**Address:** Trinitas Regional Medical Center
225 Williamson St, Elizabeth, NJ 07207
**Phone:** (908) 994-5420
**Fax:** (908) 351-7930
**Percentage of IMGs in the program:** 100%
**Minimum USMLE Step 1 Score Requirement:** No limits set
**Minimum USMLE Step 2 Score Requirement:** No limits set
**Attempts on any step:** No limits set
**CS required at time of application:** Yes including ECFMG certificate
**USCE Requirement:** None
**Cut-Off time since graduation:** No limits set
**Program offers couple match:** Yes

**Visas Sponsored or accepted:** J1 visa and H1b visa

## Newark Beth Israel Medical Center Internal Medicine Residency Program

**Specialty:** Internal Medicine
**Program name:** Newark Beth Israel Medical Center Program
**Program code:** 140-33-21-518
**NRMP Code:** 1397140M0, 1397140P0, 1397140C0
**Program type:** Community-based university affiliated hospital
**State:** New Jersey
**Address:** Newark Beth Israel Medical Center, 201 Lyons Ave, Newark, NJ 07112
**Phone:** (973) 926-7425
**Fax:** (973) 926-6130
**Percentage of IMGs in the program:** 80%
**Minimum USMLE Step 1 Score Requirement:** No limits set
**Minimum USMLE Step 2 Score Requirement:** No limits set
**Attempts on any step:** Must pass on first attempt
**CS required at time of application:** Yes
**USCE Requirement:** None
**Cut-Off time since graduation:** 3 years

**Program offers couple match:** Yes
**Visas Sponsored or accepted:** No visa

# New York Medical College at St Joseph's Regional Medical Center Internal Medicine Residency Program

**Specialty:** Internal Medicine
**Program name:** New York Medical College at St Joseph's Regional Medical Center Program
**Program code:** 140-33-21-522
**NRMP Code:** 1406140C1
**Program type:** Community-based university affiliated hospital
**State:** New Jersey
**Address:** St Joseph's Regional Medical Center
703 Main St, Paterson, NJ  07503
**Phone:** (973) 754-2431
**Fax:** (973) 754-3376
**Percentage of IMGs in the program:** 90%
**Minimum USMLE Step 1 Score Requirement:** No limits set
**Minimum USMLE Step 2 Score Requirement:** No limits set
**Attempts on any step:** No limits set
**CS required at time of application:** Yes including ECFMG certificate
**USCE Requirement:** None
**Cut-Off time since graduation:** No limits set

**Program offers couple match:** Yes
**Visas Sponsored or accepted:** J1 visa

## Drexel University College of Medicine/St Peter's University Hospital Internal Medicine Residency Program

**Specialty:** Internal Medicine
**Program name:** Drexel University College of Medicine/St Peter's University Hospital Program
**Program code:** 140-33-21-531
**NRMP Code:** 3211140C0
**Program type:** University-based
**State:** New Jersey
**Address:** St Peter's University Hospital,
          254 Easton Ave, New Brunswick, NJ 08901
**Phone:** (732) 745-8600    Ext:  8345
**Fax:** (732) 745-0406
**Percentage of IMGs in the program:** 90%
**Minimum USMLE Step 1 Score Requirement:** No limits set
**Minimum USMLE Step 2 Score Requirement:** No limits set
**Attempts on any step:** Must pass on first attempt
**CS required at time of application:** No
**USCE Requirement:** None
**Cut-Off time since graduation:** No limits set

**Program offers couple match:** Yes
**Visas Sponsored or accepted:** J1 visa and H1b visa

## AtlantiCare Regional Medical Center Internal Medicine Residency Program

**Specialty:** Internal Medicine
**Program name:** AtlantiCare Regional Medical Center Program
**Program code:** 140-33-31-226
**NRMP Code:** 1378140C0
**Program type:** Community-based
**State:** New Jersey
**Address:** AtlantiCare Regional Medical Center, 1925 Pacific Ave, Atlantic City, NJ 08401
**Phone:** (609) 441-8990
**Fax:** (609) 441-8907
**Percentage of IMGs in the program:** 90%
**Minimum USMLE Step 1 Score Requirement:** 213
**Minimum USMLE Step 2 Score Requirement:** 213
**Attempts on any step:** No limits set
**CS required at time of application:** No
**USCE Requirement:** None
**Cut-Off time since graduation:** No limits set

**Program offers couple match:** Yes
**Visas Sponsored or accepted:** J1 visa

## New Mexico

### University of New Mexico Internal Medicine Residency Program

**Specialty:** Internal Medicine
**Program name:** University of New Mexico
Program
**Program code:** 140-34-21-247
**NRMP Code:** 1962140P1, 1962140C0,
1962140P0
**Program type:** University-based
**State:** New Mexico
**Address:** University of New Mexico HSC
        1 Univ of New Mexico, Albuquerque,
NM  87131-0001
**Phone:** (505) 272-6331
**Fax:** (505) 272-4628
**Percentage of IMGs in the program:** 20%
**Minimum USMLE Step 1 Score Requirement:**
220

**Minimum USMLE Step 2 Score Requirement:**
220
**Attempts on any step:** No limits set
**CS required at time of application:** Yes
including ECFMG certificate
**USCE Requirement:** Yes, 2 months
**Cut-Off time since graduation:** 3 years
**Program offers couple match:** Yes
**Visas Sponsored or accepted:** J1 visa

# New York

## Lutheran Family Health Center Internal Medicine Residency Program

**Specialty:** Internal Medicine
**Program name:** Lutheran Family Health Center
Program
**Program code:** 140-35-00-921
**State:** New York
**Address:** Lutheran Family Health Center, Station
3-04
        150 55th St, Brooklyn, NY  11220
**Phone:** (718) 630-6374

**Fax:** (718) 630-8471
**Percentage of IMGs in the program:** 70%
**Minimum USMLE Step 1 Score Requirement:** 210
**Minimum USMLE Step 2 Score Requirement:** 210
**Attempts on any step:** Must pass on first attempt
**CS required at time of application:** Yes including ECFMG certificate
**USCE Requirement:** None
**Cut-Off time since graduation:** 5 years unless in residency or other special clinical status
**Program offers couple match:** Yes
**Visas Sponsored or accepted:** J1 visa

## University Hospital-SUNY at Stony Brook/Mather Hospital Internal Medicine Residency Program

**Specialty:** Internal Medicine
**Program name:** University Hospital-SUNY at Stony Brook/Mather Hospital Program
**Program code:** 140-35-00-922
**State:** New York
**Address:** John T Mather Memorial Hospital, Internal Medicine Program
          75 N Country Rd, Port Jefferson, NY 11777
**Phone:** (631) 686-7997

**Fax:** (631) 686-7653
**Percentage of IMGs in the program:** 50%
**Minimum USMLE Step 1 Score Requirement:**
No limits set
**Minimum USMLE Step 2 Score Requirement:**
No limits set
**Attempts on any step:** No limits set
**CS required at time of application:** Yes
including ECFMG certificate
**USCE Requirement:** None
**Cut-Off time since graduation:** 5 years
**Program offers couple match:** Yes
**Visas Sponsored or accepted:** No visa

## Bassett Medical Center Internal Medicine Residency Program

**Specialty:** Internal Medicine
**Program name:** Bassett Medical Center
Program
**Program code:** 140-35-11-253
**NRMP Code:** 1442140C0, 1442140P0,
1442140M0
**Program type:** Community-based university
affiliated hospital
**State:** New York
**Address:** Mary Imogene Bassett Hospital, Office
of Medical Education,
One Atwell Rd, Cooperstown, NY

13326-1394
**Phone:** (888) 547-6349
**Fax:** (607) 547-6612
**Percentage of IMGs in the program:** 20%
**Minimum USMLE Step 1 Score Requirement:** 205
**Minimum USMLE Step 2 Score Requirement:** 205
**Attempts on any step:** Must pass on first attempt
**CS required at time of application:** No
**USCE Requirement:** Yes
**Cut-Off time since graduation:** 4 years
**Program offers couple match:** Yes
**Visas Sponsored or accepted:** J1 visa

## Winthrop-University Hospital Internal Medicine Residency Program

**Specialty:** Internal Medicine
**Program name:** Winthrop-University Hospital Program
**Program code:** 140-35-11-256
**NRMP Code:** 1455140C0, 1455140P0
**Program type:** Community-based university affiliated hospital
**State:** New York
**Address:** Winthrop-University Hospital, Department of Medicine Suite 509,

222 Station Plaza N, Mineola, NY 11501
**Phone:** (516) 663-2781
**Fax:** (516) 663-8796
**Percentage of IMGs in the program:** 30%
**Minimum USMLE Step 1 Score Requirement:** 205
**Minimum USMLE Step 2 Score Requirement:** 205
**Attempts on any step:** Must pass on first attempt including CS exam
**CS required at time of application:** Yes including ECFMG certificate
**USCE Requirement:** None
**Cut-Off time since graduation:** No limits set
**Program offers couple match:** Yes
**Visas Sponsored or accepted:** J1 visa and H1b visa

# New York Medical College (Sound Shore) Internal Medicine Residency Program

**Specialty:** Internal Medicine
**Program name:** New York Medical College (Sound Shore) Program
**Program code:** 140-35-11-258
**State:** New York
**Address:** Sound Shore Medical Center Westchester, Internal Medicine Program,

16 Guion Pl, New Rochelle, NY  10802
**Phone:** (914) 365-3681
**Fax:** (914) 365-5489
**Percentage of IMGs in the program:** 60%
**Minimum USMLE Step 1 Score Requirement:** 215
**Minimum USMLE Step 2 Score Requirement:** 215
**Attempts on any step:** Must pass on first attempt
**CS required at time of application:** Yes including ECFMG certificate
**USCE Requirement:** None
**Cut-Off time since graduation:** No limits set
**Program offers couple match:** Yes
**Visas Sponsored or accepted:** J1 visa and H1b visa

## Albert Einstein College of Medicine at Beth Israel Medical Center Internal Medicine Residency Program

**Specialty:** Internal Medicine
**Program name:** Albert Einstein College of Medicine at Beth Israel Medical Center Program
**Program code:** 140-35-11-261
**NRMP Code:** 1470140P0, 1470140P1, 1470140C0, 1470140C2

**Program type:** University-based
**State:** New York
**Address:** Beth Israel Med Center, Department of Medicine,
First Ave at 16th St, New York, NY 10003
**Phone:** (212) 420-4012
**Fax:** (212) 420-4615
**Percentage of IMGs in the program:** 30%
**Minimum USMLE Step 1 Score Requirement:** No limits set
**Minimum USMLE Step 2 Score Requirement:** No limits set
**Attempts on any step:** No limits set
**CS required at time of application:** Yes including ECFMG certificate
**USCE Requirement:** None
**Cut-Off time since graduation:** No limits set
**Program offers couple match:** Yes
**Visas Sponsored or accepted:** J1 visa and H1b visa


# New York Hospital Medical Center of Queens/Cornell University Medical College Internal Medicine Residency Program

**Specialty:** Internal Medicine

**Program name:** New York Hospital Medical Center of Queens/Cornell University Medical College Program
**Program code:** 140-35-11-262
**NRMP Code:** 1822140P0, 1822140C0
**Program type:** Community-based university affiliated hospital
**State:** New York
**Address:** New York Hospital Queens, Department of Medicine, 5th Floor,
        56-45 Main St, Flushing, NY 11355-2966
**Phone:** (718) 670-1347
**Fax:** (718) 670-2456
**Percentage of IMGs in the program:** 30%
**Minimum USMLE Step 1 Score Requirement:** 205
**Minimum USMLE Step 2 Score Requirement:** 205
**Attempts on any step:** Must pass maximum on 2nd attempt
**CS required at time of application:** Yes including ECFMG certificate
**USCE Requirement:** None
**Cut-Off time since graduation:** 4 years
**Program offers couple match:** Yes
**Visas Sponsored or accepted:** J1 visa

# Bronx-Lebanon Hospital Center Internal Medicine Residency Program

**Specialty:** Internal Medicine
**Program name:** Bronx-Lebanon Hospital Center Program
**Program code:** 140-35-11-263
**Program type:** Community-based University affiliated hospital
**State:** New York
**Address:** Bronx-Lebanon Hospital Center, Department of Internal Medicine,
        1650 Selwyn Ave, Bronx, NY  10457
**Phone:** (718) 960-2099
**Fax:** (718) 960-2055
**Percentage of IMGs in the program:** 100%
**Minimum USMLE Step 1 Score Requirement:** 220
**Minimum USMLE Step 2 Score Requirement:** 220
**Attempts on any step:** Must pass on first attempt including CS exam
**CS required at time of application:** Yes including ECFMG certificate
**USCE Requirement:** None
**Cut-Off time since graduation:** 5 years
**Program offers couple match:** Yes
**Visas Sponsored or accepted:** J1 visa and H1b visa

# Brookdale University Hospital and Medical Center Internal Medicine Residency Program

**Specialty:** Internal Medicine
**Program name:** Brookdale University Hospital and Medical Center Program
**Program code:** 140-35-11-264
**State:** New York
**Address:** Brookdale University Hospital and Medical Center, Suite 134 CHC
One Brookdale Plaza, Brooklyn, NY 11212
**Phone:** (718) 240-6347
**Fax:** (718) 240-6516
**Percentage of IMGs in the program:** 80%
**Minimum USMLE Step 1 Score Requirement:** 220
**Minimum USMLE Step 2 Score Requirement:** 220
**Attempts on any step:** Must pass on first attempt
**CS required at time of application:** No
**USCE Requirement:** None
**Cut-Off time since graduation:** No limits set
**Program offers couple match:** Yes
**Visas Sponsored or accepted:** J1 visa

# Icahn School of Medicine at Mount Sinai (Elmhurst) Internal Medicine Residency Program

**Specialty:** Internal Medicine
**Program name:** Icahn School of Medicine at Mount Sinai (Elmhurst) Program
**Program code:** 140-35-11-268
**NRMP Code:** 1491140M0, 1491140P0
**Program type:** Community-based university affiliated hospital
**State:** New York
**Address:** Elmhurst Hospital Center-Mount Sinai, Room A1-16
          79-01 Broadway, Elmhurst, NY  11373
**Phone:** (718) 334-2490
**Fax:** (718) 334-5845
**Percentage of IMGs in the program:** 80%
**Minimum USMLE Step 1 Score Requirement:** No limits set
**Minimum USMLE Step 2 Score Requirement:** No limits set
**Attempts on any step:** No limits set
**CS required at time of application:** Yes
**USCE Requirement:** None
**Cut-Off time since graduation:** No limits set
**Program offers couple match:** Yes
**Visas Sponsored or accepted:** No visa

# Coney Island Hospital Internal Medicine Residency Program

**Specialty:** Internal Medicine
**Program name:** Coney Island Hospital Program
**Program code:** 140-35-11-269
**State:** New York
**Address:** Coney Island Hospital, Suite 4N98
2601 Ocean Pkwy, Brooklyn, NY 11235
**Phone:** (718) 616-3779
**Fax:** (718) 616-3797
**Percentage of IMGs in the program:** 100%
**Minimum USMLE Step 1 Score Requirement:** 204
**Minimum USMLE Step 2 Score Requirement:** 204
**Attempts on any step:** Must pass on first attempt
**CS required at time of application:** No
**USCE Requirement:** None
**Cut-Off time since graduation:** 5 years
**Program offers couple match:** Yes
**Visas Sponsored or accepted:** No visa

# Flushing Hospital Medical Center Internal Medicine Residency Program

**Specialty:** Internal Medicine
**Program name:** Flushing Hospital Medical Center Program
**Program code:** 140-35-11-272
**NRMP Code:** 1445140P0, 1445140C0
**Program type:** Community-based
**State:** New York
**Address:** Flushing Hospital Medical Center, Department of Medicine
        4500 Parsons Blvd, Flushing, NY  11355
**Phone:** (718) 670-5939
**Fax:** (718) 670-4510
**Percentage of IMGs in the program:** 80%
**Minimum USMLE Step 1 Score Requirement:** 205
**Minimum USMLE Step 2 Score Requirement:** 205
**Attempts on any step:** Must pass on first attempt
**CS required at time of application:** No
**USCE Requirement:** None
**Cut-Off time since graduation:** 5 years
**Program offers couple match:** Yes
**Visas Sponsored or accepted:** No visa

# Harlem Hospital Center Internal Medicine Residency Program

**Specialty:** Internal Medicine
**Program name:** Harlem Hospital Center Program
**Program code:** 140-35-11-273
**NRMP Code:** 1478140C0
**Program type:** Community-based university affiliated hospital
**State:** New York
**Address:** Harlem Hospital Center, Department of Internal Medicine

  506 Lenox Ave, New York, NY  10037
**Phone:** (212) 939-2291
**Fax:** (212) 939-2263
**Percentage of IMGs in the program:** 100%
**Minimum USMLE Step 1 Score Requirement:** 205
**Minimum USMLE Step 2 Score Requirement:** 205
**Attempts on any step:** Must pass on first attempt
**CS required at time of application:** No
**USCE Requirement:** None
**Cut-Off time since graduation:** 5 years
**Program offers couple match:** No
**Visas Sponsored or accepted:** J1 visa and H1b visa

# Kingsbrook Jewish Medical Center Internal Medicine Residency Program

**Specialty:** Internal Medicine
**Program name:** Kingsbrook Jewish Medical Center Program
**Program code:** 140-35-11-277
**NRMP Code:** 1476140C0
**Program type:** Community-based
**State:** New York
**Address:** Kingsbrook Jewish Medical Center, Department of Medicine K4,
        585 Schenectady Ave, Brooklyn, NY 11203
**Phone:** (718) 363-6771
**Fax:** (718) 604-5450
**Percentage of IMGs in the program:** 100%
**Minimum USMLE Step 1 Score Requirement:** 235
**Minimum USMLE Step 2 Score Requirement:** 235
**Attempts on any step:** Must pass on first attempt
**CS required at time of application:** Yes including ECFMG certificate
**USCE Requirement:** None
**Cut-Off time since graduation:** No limits set
**Program offers couple match:** No
**Visas Sponsored or accepted:** No visa

## NSLIJ/Hofstra North Shore-LIJ School of Medicine at Lenox Hill Hospital Internal Medicine Residency Program

**Specialty:** Internal Medicine
**Program name:** NSLIJ/Hofstra North Shore-LIJ School of Medicine at Lenox Hill Hospital Program
**Program code:** 140-35-11-278
**NRMP Code:** 1700140C2, 1700140M0, 1700140P2
**Program type:** Community-based university affiliated hospital
**State:** New York
**Address:** Lenox Hill Hospital, Department of Medicine
        100 E 77th St, New York, NY  10075
**Phone:** (212) 434-2422
**Fax:** (212) 434-2246
**Percentage of IMGs in the program:** 40%
**Minimum USMLE Step 1 Score Requirement:** No limits set
**Minimum USMLE Step 2 Score Requirement:** No limits set
**Attempts on any step:** No limits set
**CS required at time of application:** No
**USCE Requirement:** None

**Cut-Off time since graduation:** 3 years
**Program offers couple match:** Yes
**Visas Sponsored or accepted:** J1 visa

## Lutheran Medical Center Internal Medicine Residency Program

**Specialty:** Internal Medicine
**Program name:** Lutheran Medical Center Program
**Program code:** 140-35-11-282
**NRMP Code:** 1430140C0
**Program type:** Community-based university affiliated hospital
**State:** New York
**Address:** Lutheran Medical Center, Department of Medicine,
        150 55th St, Brooklyn, NY 11220
**Phone:** (718) 630-6373
**Fax:** (718) 210-2409
**Percentage of IMGs in the program:** 100%
**Minimum USMLE Step 1 Score Requirement:** 210
**Minimum USMLE Step 2 Score Requirement:** 210
**Attempts on any step:** Must pass on first attempt
**CS required at time of application:** Yes
**USCE Requirement:** None

**Cut-Off time since graduation:** 5 years
**Program offers couple match:** No
**Visas Sponsored or accepted:** No visa

## Maimonides Medical Center Internal Medicine Residency Program

**Specialty:** Internal Medicine
**Program name:** Maimonides Medical Center Program
**Program code:** 140-35-11-283
**State:** New York
**Address:** Maimonides Medical Center, Department of Medicine
4802 Tenth Ave, Brooklyn, NY  11219
**Phone:** (718) 283-8997
**Fax:** (718) 283-8498
**Percentage of IMGs in the program:** 80%
**Minimum USMLE Step 1 Score Requirement:** No limits set
**Minimum USMLE Step 2 Score Requirement:** No limits set
**Attempts on any step:** Must pass on first attempt
**CS required at time of application:** Yes including ECFMG certificate
**USCE Requirement:** None
**Cut-Off time since graduation:** 3 years

**Program offers couple match:** Yes
**Visas Sponsored or accepted:** J1 visa and H1b visa

## New York Methodist Hospital Internal Medicine Residency Program

**Specialty:** Internal Medicine
**Program name:** New York Methodist Hospital Program
**Program code:** 140-35-11-284
**NRMP Code:** 1429140C0, 1429140M0
**Program type:** Community-based university affiliated hospital
**State:** New York
**Address:** New York Methodist Hospital, Department of Medicine,
             506 Sixth St, Brooklyn, NY  11215
**Phone:** (718) 780-7343
**Fax:** (718) 780-3259
**Percentage of IMGs in the program:** 100%
**Minimum USMLE Step 1 Score Requirement:** No limits set
**Minimum USMLE Step 2 Score Requirement:** No limits set
**Attempts on any step:** No limits set
**CS required at time of application:** Yes including ECFMG certificate

**USCE Requirement:** None
**Cut-Off time since graduation:** 5 years
**Program offers couple match:** No
**Visas Sponsored or accepted:** No visa

## New York Presbyterian Hospital (Columbia Campus) Internal Medicine Residency Program

**Specialty:** Internal Medicine
**Program name:** New York Presbyterian Hospital (Columbia Campus) Program
**Program code:** 140-35-11-297
**NRMP Code:** 1495140C0
**State:** New York
**Address:** New York Presbyterian Hospital-Columbia, 6th Floor Center 12,
         177 Fort Washington Ave, New York, NY  10032
**Phone:** (212) 305-2913
**Percentage of IMGs in the program:** 5%
**Minimum USMLE Step 1 Score Requirement:** No limits set
**Minimum USMLE Step 2 Score Requirement:** No limits set
**Attempts on any step:** No limits set
**CS required at time of application:** No
**USCE Requirement:** Yes at least 1 month
**Cut-Off time since graduation:** No limits set

**Program offers couple match:** Yes
**Visas Sponsored or accepted:** J1 visa

# Richmond University Medical Center Internal Medicine Residency Program

**Specialty:** Internal Medicine
**Program name:** Richmond University Medical Center Program
**Program code:** 140-35-11-303
**State:** New York
**Address:** Richmond University Medical Center, Department of Medicine,

      355 Bard Ave, Staten Island, NY  10310
**Phone:** (718) 818-2419
**Fax:** (718) 818-3225
**Percentage of IMGs in the program:** 40%
**Minimum USMLE Step 1 Score Requirement:** 225
**Minimum USMLE Step 2 Score Requirement:** 225
**Attempts on any step:** Must pass on first attempt
**CS required at time of application:** No
**USCE Requirement:** None
**Cut-Off time since graduation:** No limits set
**Program offers couple match:** Yes
**Visas Sponsored or accepted:** J1 visa

# Staten Island University Hospital Internal Medicine Residency Program

**Specialty:** Internal Medicine
**Program name:** Staten Island University Hospital Program
**Program code:** 140-35-11-304
**NRMP Code:** 1515140P0, 1515140M0
**Program type:** Community-based university affiliated hospital
**State:** New York
**Address:** Staten Island University Hospital, Internal Medicine Program,
          475 Seaview Ave, Staten Island, NY 10305
**Phone:** (718) 226-6205
**Fax:** (718) 226-6586
**Percentage of IMGs in the program:** 60%
**Minimum USMLE Step 1 Score Requirement:** No limits set
**Minimum USMLE Step 2 Score Requirement:** No limits set
**Attempts on any step:** Must pass on first attempt (2nd attempt max on CS exam)
**CS required at time of application:** No
**USCE Requirement:** None
**Cut-Off time since graduation:** 4 years

**Program offers couple match:** Yes
**Visas Sponsored or accepted:** J1 visa and H1b visa

# New York Medical College at Westchester Medical Center Internal Medicine Residency Program

**Specialty:** Internal Medicine
**Program name:** New York Medical College at Westchester Medical Center Program
**Program code:** 140-35-11-317
**NRMP Code:** 2998140C0, 2998140P0
**Program type:** University-based
**State:** New York
**Address:** NYMC Westchester Medical Center, Department of Medicine,
          Munger Pavilion Room 253, Valhalla, NY  10595
**Phone:** (914) 493-8373
**Percentage of IMGs in the program:** 20%
**Minimum USMLE Step 1 Score Requirement:** 225
**Minimum USMLE Step 2 Score Requirement:** 225

**Attempts on any step:** Must pass on 1st attempt on step 1 and maximum on 2nd attempt on step 2
**CS required at time of application:** No
**USCE Requirement:** None
**Cut-Off time since graduation:** 2 years unless in residency or clinically active
**Program offers couple match:** Yes
**Visas Sponsored or accepted:** J1 visa and H1b visa

## Brooklyn Hospital Center Internal Medicine Residency Program

**Specialty:** Internal Medicine
**Program name:** Brooklyn Hospital Center Program
**Program code:** 140-35-12-265
**State:** New York
**Address:** Brooklyn Hospital Center, Internal Medicine Department
          121 Dekalb Ave, Brooklyn, NY  11201
**Phone:** (718) 250-6946
**Fax:** (718) 250-8120
**Percentage of IMGs in the program:** 100%
**Minimum USMLE Step 1 Score Requirement:** No limits set
**Minimum USMLE Step 2 Score Requirement:** No limits set

**Attempts on any step:** Must pass maximum on 2nd attempt
**CS required at time of application:** Yes including ECFMG certificate
**USCE Requirement:** None
**Cut-Off time since graduation:** 5 years
**Program offers couple match:** Yes
**Visas Sponsored or accepted:** No visa

## Jamaica Hospital Medical Center Internal Medicine Residency Program

**Specialty:** Internal Medicine
**Program name:** Jamaica Hospital Medical Center Program
**Program code:** 140-35-12-275
**State:** New York
**Address:** Jamaica Hospital Medical Center, Department of Medicine
8900 Van Wyck Expwy, Jamaica, NY 11418
**Phone:** (718) 206-6768
**Fax:** (718) 206-6651
**Percentage of IMGs in the program:** 100%
**Minimum USMLE Step 1 Score Requirement:** No limits set
**Minimum USMLE Step 2 Score Requirement:** No limits set
**Attempts on any step:** No limits set

**CS required at time of application:** Yes including ECFMG certificate
**USCE Requirement:** Yes at least 1 month within the last 2 years
**Cut-Off time since graduation:** 5 years
**Program offers couple match:** No
**Visas Sponsored or accepted:** J1 visa

## University at Buffalo (Catholic Health System-Sisters of Charity) Internal Medicine Residency Program

**Specialty:** Internal Medicine
**Program name:** University at Buffalo (Catholic Health System-Sisters of Charity) Program
**Program code:** 140-35-21-251
**NRMP Code:** 3099140C5, 3099140P4
**Program type:** Community-based university affiliated hospital
**State:** New York
**Address:** Sisters of Charity Hospital, Department of Medicine,
        2157 Main St, Buffalo, NY  14214
**Phone:** (716) 862-1423
**Fax:** (716) 862-1867
**Percentage of IMGs in the program:** 90%
**Minimum USMLE Step 1 Score Requirement:** 225

**Minimum USMLE Step 2 Score Requirement:** 225

**Attempts on any step:** Must pass on first attempt

**CS required at time of application:** Yes including ECFMG certificate

**USCE Requirement:** None

**Cut-Off time since graduation:** 5 years

**Program offers couple match:** Yes

**Visas Sponsored or accepted:** J1 visa

## Nassau University Medical Center Internal Medicine Residency Program

**Specialty:** Internal Medicine

**Program name:** Nassau University Medical Center Program

**Program code:** 140-35-21-254

**State:** New York

**Address:** Nassau University Medical Center, Department of Medicine

2201 Hempstead Trnpk, East Meadow, NY  11554

**Phone:** (516) 572-4835

**Fax:** (516) 572-5609

**Percentage of IMGs in the program:** 70%

**Minimum USMLE Step 1 Score Requirement:** 210

**Minimum USMLE Step 2 Score Requirement:**
210
**Attempts on any step:** Must pass on first
attempt
**CS required at time of application:** No
**USCE Requirement:** None
**Cut-Off time since graduation:** 5 years
**Program offers couple match:** Yes
**Visas Sponsored or accepted:** J1 visa

## New York Presbyterian Hospital (Cornell Campus) Internal Medicine Residency Program

**Specialty:** Internal Medicine
**Program name:** New York Presbyterian Hospital
(Cornell Campus) Program
**Program code:** 140-35-21-270
**State:** New York
**Address:** New York Presbyterian Hospital-
Cornell,

Department of Medicine Box 130 Rm
M-528,

525 E 68th St, New York, NY 10065
**Phone:** (212) 746-4749
**Fax:** (212) 746-6692
**Percentage of IMGs in the program:** 10%
**Minimum USMLE Step 1 Score Requirement:**
No limits set

**Minimum USMLE Step 2 Score Requirement:**
No limits set
**Attempts on any step:** No limits set
**CS required at time of application:** Yes
including ECFMG certificate
**USCE Requirement:** None
**Cut-Off time since graduation:** No limits set
**Program offers couple match:** Yes
**Visas Sponsored or accepted:** J1 visa

## Interfaith Medical Center Internal Medicine Residency Program

**Specialty:** Internal Medicine
**Program name:** Interfaith Medical Center
Program
**Program code:** 140-35-21-276
**NRMP Code:** 1425140M0
**Program type:** Community-based
**State:** New York
**Address:** Interfaith Medical Center, Department
of Medicine,
          1545 Atlantic Ave, Brooklyn, NY
11213
**Phone:** (718) 613-4063
**Fax:** (718) 613-4893
**Percentage of IMGs in the program:** 100%
**Minimum USMLE Step 1 Score Requirement:**
220

**Minimum USMLE Step 2 Score Requirement:** 220
**Attempts on any step:** Must pass on first attempt
**CS required at time of application:** Yes including ECFMG certificate
**USCE Requirement:** None
**Cut-Off time since graduation:** No limits set
**Program offers couple match:** Yes
**Visas Sponsored or accepted:** J1 visa and H1b visa

## NSLIJHS/Hofstra North Shore-LIJ School of Medicine Internal Medicine Residency Program

**Specialty:** Internal Medicine
**Program name:** NSLIJHS/Hofstra North Shore-LIJ School of Medicine Program
**Program code:** 140-35-21-281
**NRMP Code:** 1700140C0, 1700140P0
**Program type:** University-based
**State:** New York
**Address:** Long Island Jewish Medical Center, Department of Medicine 2nd Floor,
270-05 76th Ave, New Hyde Park, NY 11040
**Phone:** (516) 562-4764

**Fax:**
**Percentage of IMGs in the program:** 10%
**Minimum USMLE Step 1 Score Requirement:**
No limits set
**Minimum USMLE Step 2 Score Requirement:**
No limits set
**Attempts on any step:** No limits set
**CS required at time of application:** No
**USCE Requirement:** None
**Cut-Off time since graduation:** 3 years
**Program offers couple match:** Yes
**Visas Sponsored or accepted:** J1 visa and H1b
visa

## Albert Einstein College of Medicine Internal Medicine Residency Program

**Specialty:** Internal Medicine
**Program name:** Albert Einstein College of
Medicine Program
**Program code:** 140-35-21-285
**NRMP Code:** 1486140C0
**Program type:** Community-based university
affiliated hospital
**State:** New York
**Address:** Montefiore Medical Center-Wakefield
Campus,

Department of Medicine 5th Floor,
600 E 233rd St, Bronx, NY  10466

**Phone**: (718) 920-9880

**Percentage of IMGs in the program:** 100%

**Minimum USMLE Step 1 Score Requirement:** No limits set

**Minimum USMLE Step 2 Score Requirement:** No limits set

**Attempts on any step:** No limits set

**CS required at time of application:** Yes including ECFMG certificate

**USCE Requirement:** None

**Cut-Off time since graduation:** 3 years

**Program offers couple match:** No

**Visas Sponsored or accepted:** J1 visa and H1b visa

## Albert Einstein College of Medicine (Montefiore) Internal Medicine Residency Program

**Specialty:** Internal Medicine

**Program name:** Albert Einstein College of Medicine (Montefiore) Program

**Program code:** 140-35-21-287

**NRMP Code:** University-based

**Program type:** 3153140M0, 3153140C0, 3153140P1, 3153140P2, 3153140P0

**State:** New York

**Address:** Montefiore Medical Center, NW 651, 111 E 210th St, Bronx, NY  10467

**Phone:** (718) 920-4417
**Fax:** (718) 920-8375
**Percentage of IMGs in the program:** 10%
**Minimum USMLE Step 1 Score Requirement:** No limits set
**Minimum USMLE Step 2 Score Requirement:** No limits set
**Attempts on any step:** Must pass on first attempt
**CS required at time of application:** Yes including ECFMG certificate
**USCE Requirement:** None
**Cut-Off time since graduation:** 3 years
**Program offers couple match:** Yes
**Visas Sponsored or accepted:** J1 visa and H1b visa

## New York University School of Medicine Internal Medicine Residency Program

**Specialty:** Internal Medicine
**Program name:** New York University School of Medicine Program
**Program code:** 140-35-21-292
**NRMP Code:** 2978140P0, 2978140C1, 2978140M0, 2978140C0
**Program type:** University-based
**State:** New York

**Address:** New York University School of Medicine,

Department of Medicine NBV 16 N 30
550 First Ave, New York, NY 10016

**Phone:** (212) 263-6397
**Fax:** (212) 263-2913
**Percentage of IMGs in the program:** 5%
**Minimum USMLE Step 1 Score Requirement:** No limits set
**Minimum USMLE Step 2 Score Requirement:** No limits set
**Attempts on any step:** No limits set
**CS required at time of application:** No
**USCE Requirement:** Yes
**Cut-Off time since graduation:** 5 years
**Program offers couple match:** Yes
**Visas Sponsored or accepted:** J1 visa and H1b visa

# Icahn School of Medicine at Mount Sinai/St Luke's-Roosevelt Hospital Center Internal Medicine Residency Program

**Specialty:** Internal Medicine
**Program name:** Icahn School of Medicine at Mount Sinai/St Luke's-Roosevelt Hospital Center Program
**Program code:** 140-35-21-301

**NRMP Code:** 2070140P0, 2070140C0
**Program type:** Community-based university affiliated hospital
**State:** New York
**Address:** St Luke's-Roosevelt Hospital/Mount Sinai Care System,

Department of Medicine 3rd Floor Suite 3A-02,

1000 10th Ave, New York, NY  10019
**Phone:** (212) 523-7321
**Fax:** (212) 523-8605
**Percentage of IMGs in the program:** 70%
**Minimum USMLE Step 1 Score Requirement:** No limits set
**Minimum USMLE Step 2 Score Requirement:** No limits set
**Attempts on any step:** Must pass on first attempt
**CS required at time of application:** Yes including ECFMG certificate
**USCE Requirement:** None but must be clinically active within the past 2 years
**Cut-Off time since graduation:** 5 years
**Program offers couple match:** Yes
**Visas Sponsored or accepted:** J1 visa and H1b visa

## SUNY Health Science Center at Brooklyn Internal Medicine Residency Program

**Specialty:** Internal Medicine
**Program name:** SUNY Health Science Center at Brooklyn Program
**Program code:** 140-35-21-305
**NRMP Code:** 1426140P0, 1426140C0
**Program type:** University-based
**State:** New York
**Address:** SUNY Downstate Medical Center, Department of Medicine Box 50,
         450 Clarkson Ave, Brooklyn, NY  11203
**Phone:** (718) 270-2353
**Fax:** (718) 270-4488
**Percentage of IMGs in the program:** 40%
**Minimum USMLE Step 1 Score Requirement:** 210
**Minimum USMLE Step 2 Score Requirement:** 210
**Attempts on any step:** Must pass on first attempt
**CS required at time of application:** Yes including ECFMG certificate
**USCE Requirement:** None
**Cut-Off time since graduation:** 5 years
**Program offers couple match:** Yes
**Visas Sponsored or accepted:** J1 visa and H1b visa

## SUNY at Stony Brook Internal Medicine Residency Program

**Specialty:** Internal Medicine
**Program name:** SUNY at Stony Brook Program
**Program code:** 140-35-21-315
**NRMP Code:** 2919140C0, 2919140P0, 2919140M0
**Program type:** University-based
**State:** New York
**Address:** SUNY Stony Brook University, Department of Medicine,
            HSC T-16 Room 020, Stony Brook, NY 11794-8160
**Phone:** (631) 444-7411
**Fax:** (631) 444-2493
**Percentage of IMGs in the program:** 60%
**Minimum USMLE Step 1 Score Requirement:** No limits set
**Minimum USMLE Step 2 Score Requirement:** No limits set
**Attempts on any step:** No limits set
**CS required at time of application:** Yes including ECFMG certificate
**USCE Requirement:** None
**Cut-Off time since graduation:** 5 years
**Program offers couple match:** Yes
**Visas Sponsored or accepted:** No visa

## SUNY Upstate Medical University Internal Medicine Residency Program

**Specialty:** Internal Medicine
**Program name:** SUNY Upstate Medical University Program
**Program code:** 140-35-21-316
**NRMP Code:** 1516140P0, 1516140C0
**Program type:** University-based
**State:** New York
**Address:** SUNY Upstate Medical University, Room 5138,

      750 E Adams St, Syracuse, NY 13210
**Phone:** (800) 876-7925
**Fax:** (315) 464-4484
**Percentage of IMGs in the program:** 80%
**Minimum USMLE Step 1 Score Requirement:** 220
**Minimum USMLE Step 2 Score Requirement:** 220
**Attempts on any step:** Must pass on first attempt
**CS required at time of application:** Yes including ECFMG certificate
**USCE Requirement:** None
**Cut-Off time since graduation:** No limits set
**Program offers couple match:** Yes

**Visas Sponsored or accepted:** J1 visa

## NSLIJHS/Hofstra North Shore-LIJ School of Medicine at Forest Hills Internal Medicine Residency Program

**Specialty:** Internal Medicine
**Program name:** NSLIJHS/Hofstra North Shore-LIJ School of Medicine at Forest Hills Program
**Program code:** 140-35-21-468
**NRMP Code:** 1700140C1, 1700140P1
**Program type:** University-based
**State:** New York
**Address:** North Shore LIJ-Forest Hills Hospital, Department of Medicine 9th Floor 102-01 66th Rd, Forest Hills, NY 11375
**Phone:** (718) 830-4352
**Fax:** (718) 830-1015
**Percentage of IMGs in the program:** 70%
**Minimum USMLE Step 1 Score Requirement:** No limits set
**Minimum USMLE Step 2 Score Requirement:** No limits set
**Attempts on any step:** Must pass on first attempt
**CS required at time of application:** Yes including ECFMG certificate
**USCE Requirement:** None

**Cut-Off time since graduation:** 3 years
**Program offers couple match:** Yes
**Visas Sponsored or accepted:** J1 visa and H1b visa

## Lincoln Medical and Mental Health Center Internal Medicine Residency Program

**Specialty:** Internal Medicine
**Program name:** Lincoln Medical and Mental Health Center Program
**Program code:** 140-35-21-470
**NRMP Code:** 1484140P0, 1484140C0
**Program type:** Community-based
**State:** New York
**Address:** Lincoln Medical and Mental Health Center,

Department of Internal Medicine,
234 E 149th St, Bronx, NY 10993
**Phone:** (718) 579-5016
**Fax:**(718) 579-4836
**Percentage of IMGs in the program:** 90%
**Minimum USMLE Step 1 Score Requirement:** 204
**Minimum USMLE Step 2 Score Requirement:** 204
**Attempts on any step:** Must pass on first attempt

**CS required at time of application:** No
**USCE Requirement:** None
**Cut-Off time since graduation:** 10 years
**Program offers couple match:** Yes
**Visas Sponsored or accepted:** J1 visa and H1b visa

## Mount Vernon Hospital Internal Medicine Residency Program

**Specialty:** Internal Medicine
**Program name:** Mount Vernon Hospital Program
**Program code:** 140-35-21-482
**State:** New York
**Address:** Mount Vernon Hospital, Medical Education Department,
        12 N 7th Ave, Mount Vernon, NY 10550-2026
**Phone:** (914) 361-6441
**Fax:** (914) 371-1184
**Percentage of IMGs in the program:** 100%
**Minimum USMLE Step 1 Score Requirement:** No limits set
**Minimum USMLE Step 2 Score Requirement:** No limits set
**Attempts on any step:** No limits set
**CS required at time of application:** Yes including ECFMG certificate

**USCE Requirement:** None
**Cut-Off time since graduation:** No limits set
**Program offers couple match:** Yes
**Visas Sponsored or accepted:** J1 visa and H1b visa

## St Barnabas Hospital Internal Medicine Residency Program

**Specialty:** Internal Medicine
**Program name:** St Barnabas Hospital Program
**Program code:** 140-35-21-485
**NRMP Code:** 3113140C0
**Program type:** Community-based university affiliated hospital
**State:** New York
**Address:** St Barnabas Hospital, Department of Internal Med Mills Building 3rd Floor,
          4422 Third Ave, Bronx, NY  10457
**Phone:** (718) 960-6202
**Fax:** (718) 960-3486
**Percentage of IMGs in the program:** 100%
**Minimum USMLE Step 1 Score Requirement:** No limits set
**Minimum USMLE Step 2 Score Requirement:** No limits set
**Attempts on any step:** Must pass on first attempt on the written tests

**CS required at time of application:** Yes including ECFMG certificate
**USCE Requirement:** None
**Cut-Off time since graduation:** 10 years
**Program offers couple match:** Yes
**Visas Sponsored or accepted:** J1 visa and H1b visa

## St John's Episcopal Hospital-South Shore Internal Medicine Residency Program

**Specialty:** Internal Medicine
**Program name:** St John's Episcopal Hospital-South Shore Program
**Program code:** 140-35-21-486
**State:** New York
**Address:** St John's Episcopal Hospital-South Shore, Department of Medicine,
          327 Beach 19th St, Far Rockaway, NY 11691
**Phone:** (718) 869-7672
**Fax:** (718) 869-8530
**Percentage of IMGs in the program:** 100%
**Minimum USMLE Step 1 Score Requirement:** No limits set
**Minimum USMLE Step 2 Score Requirement:** No limits set
**Attempts on any step:** No limits set

**CS required at time of application:** Yes including ECFMG certificate
**USCE Requirement:** None but strongly preferred
**Cut-Off time since graduation:** No limits set
**Program offers couple match:** Yes
**Visas Sponsored or accepted:** J1 visa and H1b visa

## Woodhull Medical and Mental Health Center Internal Medicine Residency Program

**Specialty:** Internal Medicine
**Program name:** Woodhull Medical and Mental Health Center Program
**Program code:** 140-35-21-487
**NRMP Code:** 3116140P0, 3116140M0
**Program type:** Community-based university affiliated hospital
**State:** New York
**Address:** Woodhull Medical and Mental Health Center, Department of Internal Medicine,
            760 Broadway, Brooklyn, NY 11206
**Phone:** (718) 963-5807
**Fax:** (718) 963-8753
**Percentage of IMGs in the program:** 100%
**Minimum USMLE Step 1 Score Requirement:** No limits set

**Minimum USMLE Step 2 Score Requirement:** No limits set
**Attempts on any step:** No limits set
**CS required at time of application:** No
**USCE Requirement:** None
**Cut-Off time since graduation:** 5 years
**Program offers couple match:** Yes
**Visas Sponsored or accepted:** J1 visa and H1b visa

## Icahn School of Medicine at Mount Sinai (Queens Hospital Center) Internal Medicine Residency Program

**Specialty:** Internal Medicine
**Program name:** Icahn School of Medicine at Mount Sinai (Queens Hospital Center) Program
**Program code:** 140-35-21-510
**NRMP Code:** 1489140C0, 1489140P0
**Program type:** Community-based university affiliated hospital
**State:** New York
**Address:** Queens Hospital Center, Department of Medicine N705,
        82-68 164th St, Jamaica, NY  11432
**Phone:** (718) 883-4080
**Fax:** (718) 883-6197
**Percentage of IMGs in the program:** 90%

**Minimum USMLE Step 1 Score Requirement:** 225
**Minimum USMLE Step 2 Score Requirement:** 225
**Attempts on any step:** Must pass on first attempt
**CS required at time of application:** Yes including ECFMG certificate
**USCE Requirement:** None
**Cut-Off time since graduation:** 4 years
**Program offers couple match:** Yes
**Visas Sponsored or accepted:** J1 visa

## Wyckoff Heights Medical Center Internal Medicine Residency Program

**Specialty:** Internal Medicine
**Program name:** Wyckoff Heights Medical Center Program
**Program code:** 140-35-21-520
**Program type:** Community-based university affiliated hospital
**State:** New York
**Address:** Wyckoff Heights Medical Center, Department of Internal Medicine,
           374 Stockholm St, Brooklyn, NY  11237
**Phone:** (718) 963-6444

**Fax:** (718) 486-4270
**Percentage of IMGs in the program:** 80%
**Minimum USMLE Step 1 Score Requirement:**
208
**Minimum USMLE Step 2 Score Requirement:**
208
**Attempts on any step:** Must pass on first
attempt
**CS required at time of application:** Yes
including ECFMG certificate
**USCE Requirement:** None
**Cut-Off time since graduation:** No limits set
**Program offers couple match:** No
**Visas Sponsored or accepted:** J1 visa and H1b
visa


## Albany Medical Center Internal Medicine Residency Program


**Specialty:** Internal Medicine
**Program name:** Albany Medical Center Program
**Program code:** 140-35-31-248
**State:** New York
**Address:** Albany Medical Center, Medical
Education Office MC 17
            47 New Scotland Ave, Albany, NY
12208
**Phone:** (518) 262-5377

**Fax:** (518) 262-6873
**Percentage of IMGs in the program:** 70%
**Minimum USMLE Step 1 Score Requirement:** 225
**Minimum USMLE Step 2 Score Requirement:** 225
**Attempts on any step:** Must pass on first attempt
**CS required at time of application:** Yes including ECFMG certificate
**USCE Requirement:** 6 months (UKCE also count)
**Cut-Off time since graduation:** 5 years
**Program offers couple match:** Yes
**Visas Sponsored or accepted:** J1 visa

## University at Buffalo Internal Medicine Residency Program

**Specialty:** Internal Medicine
**Program name:** University at Buffalo Program
**Program code:** 140-35-31-252
**NRMP Code:** 3099140C0, 3099140P0
**Program type:** University-based
**State:** New York
**Address:** Erie County Medical Center, Department of Medicine,
          462 Grider St, Buffalo, NY  14215
**Phone:** (716) 898-4806

**Fax:** (716) 898-3279
**Percentage of IMGs in the program:** 80%
**Minimum USMLE Step 1 Score Requirement:** 225
**Minimum USMLE Step 2 Score Requirement:** 225
**Attempts on any step:** Must pass on first attempt
**CS required at time of application:** No
**USCE Requirement:** None
**Cut-Off time since graduation:** 3 years
**Program offers couple match:** Yes
**Visas Sponsored or accepted:** J1 visa

## United Health Services Hospitals Internal Medicine Residency Program

**Specialty:** Internal Medicine
**Program name:** United Health Services Hospitals Program
**Program code:** 140-35-31-255
**NRMP Code:** 1452140M0, 1452140P0
**Program type:** Community-based university affiliated hospital
**State:** New York
**Address:** UHS Wilson Medical Center, Department of Internal Medicine,

33-57 Harrison St, Johnson City, NY 13790
**Phone:** (800) 338-8471
**Fax:** (607) 798-1629
**Percentage of IMGs in the program:** 80%
**Minimum USMLE Step 1 Score Requirement:** 210
**Minimum USMLE Step 2 Score Requirement:** 210
**Attempts on any step:** No limits set
**CS required at time of application:** Yes including ECFMG certificate
**USCE Requirement:** None
**Cut-Off time since graduation:** 8 years
**Program offers couple match:** Yes
**Visas Sponsored or accepted:** J1 visa and H1b visa

## New York Medical College (Metropolitan) Internal Medicine Residency Program

**Specialty:** Internal Medicine
**Program name:** New York Medical College (Metropolitan) Program
**Program code:** 140-35-31-290
**NRMP Code:** 1473140C0, 1473140P0
**State:** New York

**Address:** Metropolitan Hospital Center, Department of Medicine,
             1901 First Ave, New York, NY  10029
**Phone:** (212) 423-6771
**Fax:** (212) 423-8099
**Percentage of IMGs in the program:** 80%
**Minimum USMLE Step 1 Score Requirement:** No limits set
**Minimum USMLE Step 2 Score Requirement:** No limits set
**Attempts on any step:** No limits set
**CS required at time of application:** No
**USCE Requirement:** None
**Cut-Off time since graduation:** 5 years
**Program offers couple match:** Yes
**Visas Sponsored or accepted:** J1 visa and H1b visa

# Icahn School of Medicine at Mount Sinai (Bronx) Internal Medicine Residency Program

**Specialty:** Internal Medicine
**Program name:** Icahn School of Medicine at Mount Sinai (Bronx) Program
**Program code:** 140-35-31-517
**Program type:** Community-based university affiliated hospital
**State:** New York
**Address:** James J Peters VA Medical Center,

Room 7A-11,

130 W Kingsbridge Rd, Bronx, NY 10468

**Phone:** (718) 584-9000   Ext:  6753

**Fax:** (718) 741-4233

**Percentage of IMGs in the program:** 100% (Total pre-match is not uncommon)

**Minimum USMLE Step 1 Score Requirement:** 230

**Minimum USMLE Step 2 Score Requirement:** 230

**Attempts on any step:** Must pass on first attempt

**CS required at time of application:** Yes including ECFMG certificate

**USCE Requirement:** None

**Cut-Off time since graduation:** 5 years

**Program offers couple match:** Yes

**Visas Sponsored or accepted:** H1 visa

## Albert Einstein College of Medicine (Jacobi) Internal Medicine Residency Program

**Specialty:** Internal Medicine

**Program name:** Albert Einstein College of Medicine (Jacobi) Program

**Program code:** 140-35-31-521

**NRMP Code:**  3172140P0, 3172140M0,

3172140C0, 3172140C1
**Program type:** University-based
**State:** New York
**Address:** Jacobi Medical Center, Department of
Internal Medicine,
       1400 Pelham Pkwy S, Bronx, NY  10461
**Phone:** (718) 918-5642
**Fax:** (718) 918-7460
**Percentage of IMGs in the program:** 50%
**Minimum USMLE Step 1 Score Requirement:**
220
**Minimum USMLE Step 2 Score Requirement:**
220
**Attempts on any step:** No limits set
**CS required at time of application:** Yes
**USCE Requirement:** None
**Cut-Off time since graduation:** No limits set
**Program offers couple match:** Yes
**Visas Sponsored or accepted:** J1 visa and H1b
visa

## Unity Health System (Rochester) Internal Medicine Residency Program

**Specialty:** Internal Medicine
**Program name:** Unity Health System
(Rochester) Program
**Program code:** 140-35-31-527
**NRMP Code:** 1510140C0, 1510140P0

**Program type:** Community-based university affiliated hospital
**State:** New York
**Address:** Unity Health System, Department of Medicine,
1555 Long Pond Rd, Rochester, NY 14626
**Phone:** (585) 723-7775
**Fax:** (585) 723-7834
**Percentage of IMGs in the program:** 100%
**Minimum USMLE Step 1 Score Requirement:** No limits set
**Minimum USMLE Step 2 Score Requirement:** No limits set
**Attempts on any step:** No limits set
**CS required at time of application:** Yes
**USCE Requirement:** None
**Cut-Off time since graduation:** No limits set
**Program offers couple match:** No
**Visas Sponsored or accepted:** J1 visa and H1b visa

# North Carolina

## Moses H Cone Memorial Hospital Internal Medicine Residency Program

**Specialty:** Internal Medicine
**Program name:** Moses H Cone Memorial Hospital Program
**Program code:** 140-36-11-321
**NRMP Code:** 1943140C0, 1943140P0
**Program type:** Community-based university affiliated hospital
**State:** North Carolina
**Address:** Moses H Cone Memorial Hospital,
Department of Internal Medicine Suite 1006,
1200 N Elm St, Greensboro, NC 27401-1020
**Phone:** (336) 832-7800
**Fax:** (336) 832-8026
**Percentage of IMGs in the program:** 20%
**Minimum USMLE Step 1 Score Requirement:** 220
**Minimum USMLE Step 2 Score Requirement:** 220
**Attempts on any step:** Must pass on first attempt
**CS required at time of application:** No

**USCE Requirement:** 1 month
**Cut-Off time since graduation:** 5 years
**Program offers couple match:** Yes
**Visas Sponsored or accepted:** J1 visa

## Vidant Medical Center/East Carolina University Internal Medicine Residency Program

**Specialty:** Internal Medicine
**Program name:** Vidant Medical Center/East Carolina University Program
**Program code:** 140-36-11-323
**NRMP Code:** 3057140C0, 3057140P0
**Program type:** University-based
**State:** North Carolina
**Address:** Vidant Medical Center, 600 Moye Blvd, Greenville, NC 27834
**Phone:** (252) 744-3682
**Fax:** (252) 744-2280
**Percentage of IMGs in the program:** 50%
**Minimum USMLE Step 1 Score Requirement:** 205
**Minimum USMLE Step 2 Score Requirement:** 205
**Attempts on any step:** Must pass on first attempt
**CS required at time of application:** No but must pass on first attempt
**USCE Requirement:** 1 month

**Cut-Off time since graduation:** 5 years
**Program offers couple match:** Yes
**Visas Sponsored or accepted:** J1 visa


## New Hanover Regional Medical Center Internal Medicine Residents Program

**Specialty:** Internal Medicine
**Program name:** New Hanover Regional Medical Center Program
**Program code:** 140-36-11-324
**NRMP Code:** 1534140P0, 1534140C0
**Program type:** Community-based university affiliated hospital
**State:** North Carolina
**Address:** New Hanover Regional Medical Center,
            2131 S 17th St, Wilmington, NC 28402-9025
**Phone:** (910) 667-9283
**Fax:** (910) 762-6800
**Percentage of IMGs in the program:** 50%
**Minimum USMLE Step 1 Score Requirement:** 210
**Minimum USMLE Step 2 Score Requirement:** 210
**Attempts on any step:** Must pass on first attempt
**CS required at time of application:** Yes

**USCE Requirement:** Strongly preferred
**Cut-Off time since graduation:** 5 years
**Program offers couple match:** Yes
**Visas Sponsored or accepted:** No visa

## University of North Carolina Hospitals Internal Medicine Residency Program

**Specialty:** Internal Medicine
**Program name:** University of North Carolina Hospitals Program
**Program code:** 140-36-21-318
**NRMP Code:**
**Program type:**
**State:** North Carolina
**Address:** University of North Carolina Hospitals, Internal Medicine Program,
        126 Macnider Hall, CB#7005, Chapel Hill, NC  27599-7005
**Phone:** (919) 966-1216
**Fax:** (919) 843-2356
**Percentage of IMGs in the program:** 5%
**Minimum USMLE Step 1 Score Requirement:** No limits set
**Minimum USMLE Step 2 Score Requirement:** No limits set
**Attempts on any step:** No limits set
**CS required at time of application:** No
**USCE Requirement:** Yes 1 year

**Cut-Off time since graduation:** No limits set
**Program offers couple match:** Yes
**Visas Sponsored or accepted:** J1 visa

## Duke University Hospital Internal Medicine Residency Program

**Specialty:** Internal Medicine
**Program name:** Duke University Hospital Program
**Program code:** 140-36-21-320
**NRMP Code:** 1529140P1, 1529140P0, 1529140C0
**Program type:** University-based
**State:** North Carolina
**Address:** Duke University Medical Center, 2301 Erwin Rd, Durham, NC 27710
**Phone:** (919) 681-1464
**Percentage of IMGs in the program:** 5%
**Minimum USMLE Step 1 Score Requirement:** No limits set
**Minimum USMLE Step 2 Score Requirement:** No limits set
**Attempts on any step:** No limits set
**CS required at time of application:** Yes including ECFMG certificate
**USCE Requirement:** None
**Cut-Off time since graduation:** No limits set
**Program offers couple match:** Yes
**Visas Sponsored or accepted:** J1 visa

# North Dakota

## University of North Dakota Internal Medicine Residency Program

**Specialty:** Internal Medicine
**Program name:** University of North Dakota Program
**Program code:** 140-37-21-326
**NRMP Code:** 1539140C0
**Program type:** Community-based university affiliated hospital
**State:** North Dakota
**Address:** University of North Dakota School of Medicine, Medical Education Center,
      1919 N Elm St, Fargo, ND  58102
**Phone:** (701) 234-6353
**Fax:** (701) 234-7230
**Percentage of IMGs in the program:** 70%
**Minimum USMLE Step 1 Score Requirement:** No limits set
**Minimum USMLE Step 2 Score Requirement:** No limits set
**Attempts on any step:** Must pass on first

attempt
**CS required at time of application:** Yes
including ECFMG certificate
**USCE Requirement:** None
**Cut-Off time since graduation:** 3 years unless
clinically active within the past 3 years
**Program offers couple match:** Yes
**Visas Sponsored or accepted:** J1 visa and H1b
visa

# Ohio

## Summa Health System/NEOMED Internal Medicine Residency Program

**Specialty:** Internal Medicine
**Program name:** Summa Health
System/NEOMED Program
**Program code:** 140-38-11-327
**NRMP Code:** 1541140C0, 1541140P0
**Program type:** Community-based university
affiliated hospital
**State:** Ohio
**Address:** Summa Health System, Internal
Medicine Program,

525 E Market St, Akron, OH  44309
**Phone:** (330) 375-3202
**Fax:** (330) 375-3760
**Percentage of IMGs in the program:** 20%
**Minimum USMLE Step 1 Score Requirement:**
No limits set
**Minimum USMLE Step 2 Score Requirement:**
No limits set
**Attempts on any step:** Must pass on first
attempt
**CS required at time of application:** No
**USCE Requirement:** None
**Cut-Off time since graduation:** 3 years
**Program offers couple match:** Yes
**Visas Sponsored or accepted:** J1 visa

## Akron General Medical Center/NEOMED Program

**Specialty:** Internal Medicine
**Program name:** Akron General Medical
Center/NEOMED Program
**Program code:** 140-38-11-328
**NRMP Code:** 1542140C0, 1542140P0
**Program type:** Community-based university
affiliated hospital
**State:** Ohio
**Address:** Akron General Medical Center,
Department of Medicine,
400 Wabash Ave, Akron, OH  44307

**Phone:** (330) 344-6140
**Fax:** (330) 535-9270
**Percentage of IMGs in the program:** 80%
**Minimum USMLE Step 1 Score Requirement:** 225
**Minimum USMLE Step 2 Score Requirement:** 225
**Attempts on any step:** Must pass on first attempt
**CS required at time of application:** No
**USCE Requirement:** None
**Cut-Off time since graduation:** 5 years
**Program offers couple match:** Yes
**Visas Sponsored or accepted:** J1 visa

## Christ Hospital Internal Medicine Residency Program

**Specialty:** Internal Medicine
**Program name:** Christ Hospital Program
**Program code:** 140-38-11-331
**NRMP Code:** 1547140P0, 1547140C0
**Program type:** Community-based university affiliated hospital
**State:** Ohio
**Address:** Christ Hospital, Department of Medicine,
        2139 Auburn Ave, Cincinnati, OH 45219
**Phone:** (513) 585-0855

**Fax:** (513) 585-2673
**Percentage of IMGs in the program:** 40%
**Minimum USMLE Step 1 Score Requirement:** 215
**Minimum USMLE Step 2 Score Requirement:** 215
**Attempts on any step:** Must pass on first attempt
**CS required at time of application:** No
**USCE Requirement:** None
**Cut-Off time since graduation:** 5 years
**Program offers couple match:** Yes
**Visas Sponsored or accepted:** H1b visa

## Jewish Hospital of Cincinnati Internal Medicine Residency Program

**Specialty:** Internal Medicine
**Program name:** Jewish Hospital of Cincinnati Program
**Program code:** 140-38-11-333
**NRMP Code:**
**Program type:**
**State:** Ohio
**Address:** Jewish Hospital Cincinnati, Department of Internal Medicine,
         4777 E Galbraith Rd, Cincinnati, OH 45236
**Phone:** (513) 686-5441

**Fax:** (513) 686-5443
**Percentage of IMGs in the program:** 80%
**Minimum USMLE Step 1 Score Requirement:**
No limits set
**Minimum USMLE Step 2 Score Requirement:**
No limits set
**Attempts on any step:** No limits set
**CS required at time of application:** Yes
including ECFMG certificate
**USCE Requirement:** None
**Cut-Off time since graduation:** 5 years
**Program offers couple match:** Yes
**Visas Sponsored or accepted:** J1 visa and H1b
visa

## Case Western Reserve University (MetroHealth) Internal Medicine Residency Program

**Specialty:** Internal Medicine
**Program name:** Case Western Reserve
University (MetroHealth) Program
**Program code:** 140-38-11-336
**NRMP Code:** 1553140P0, 1553140C4,
1553140P1, 1553140C3, 1553140C0
**Program type:** University-based
**State:** Ohio
**Address:** MetroHealth Medical Center, Internal
Medicine Program,
        2500 MetroHealth Dr, Cleveland, OH

44109-1998
**Phone:** (216) 778-3886
**Fax:** (216) 778-5823
**Percentage of IMGs in the program:** 80%
**Minimum USMLE Step 1 Score Requirement:** 220
**Minimum USMLE Step 2 Score Requirement:** 220
**Attempts on any step:** Must pass on first attempt
**CS required at time of application:** No
**USCE Requirement:** Yes 2 months
**Cut-Off time since graduation:** 10 years
**Program offers couple match:** Yes
**Visas Sponsored or accepted:** J1 visa

## St Vincent Charity Medical Center/Case Western Reserve University Internal Medicine Residency Program

**Specialty:** Internal Medicine
**Program name:** St Vincent Charity Medical Center/Case Western Reserve University Program
**Program code:** 140-38-11-338
**NRMP Code:**
**Program type:**
**State:** Ohio
**Address:** St Vincent Charity Hospital,

Department of Internal Medicine,
        2351 E 22nd St, Cleveland, OH 44115
**Phone:** (216) 363-2725
**Fax:** (216) 363-2721
**Percentage of IMGs in the program:** 100%
**Minimum USMLE Step 1 Score Requirement:** 215
**Minimum USMLE Step 2 Score Requirement:** 215
**Attempts on any step:** Preferably, must pass on first attempt.
**CS required at time of application:** Yes including ECFMG certificate
**USCE Requirement:** None
**Cut-Off time since graduation:** No limits set
**Program offers couple match:** Yes
**Visas Sponsored or accepted:** J1 visa and H1b visa


## St Elizabeth Health Center/NEOMED Internal Medicine Residency Program

**Specialty:** Internal Medicine
**Program name:** St Elizabeth Health Center/NEOMED Program
**Program code:** 140-38-11-349
**NRMP Code:** 1584140C0
**Program type:** Community-based university

,

affiliated hospital
**State:** Ohio
**Address:** St Elizabeth Health Center, PO Box 1790,

        1044 Belmont Ave, Youngstown, OH 44501-1790
**Phone:** (330) 480-7643
**Fax:** (330) 480-3777
**Percentage of IMGs in the program:** 90%
**Minimum USMLE Step 1 Score Requirement:** No limits set
**Minimum USMLE Step 2 Score Requirement:** No limits set
**Attempts on any step:** Must pass on first attempt
**CS required at time of application:** No
**USCE Requirement:** None
**Cut-Off time since graduation:** No limits set
**Program offers couple match:** Yes


## Cleveland Clinic Foundation Internal Medicine Residency Program

**Specialty:** Internal Medicine
**Program name:** Cleveland Clinic Foundation Program
**Program code:** 140-38-12-339
**NRMP Code:** 1968140M0, 1968140C0, 1968140P0

**Program type:** Community-based university affiliated hospital
**State:** Ohio
**Address:** Cleveland Clinic, Internal Medicine Office NA-10
 9500 Euclid Ave, Cleveland, OH  44195
**Phone:** (216) 444-2336
**Fax:** (216) 445-6290
**Percentage of IMGs in the program:** 40%
**Minimum USMLE Step 1 Score Requirement:** 220
**Minimum USMLE Step 2 Score Requirement:** 220
**Attempts on any step:** Must pass on first attempt
**CS required at time of application:** Yes
**USCE Requirement:** Yes 1 year
**Cut-Off time since graduation:** No limits set
**Program offers couple match:** Yes
**Visas Sponsored or accepted:** J1 visa and H1b visa

## Mount Carmel Health System Internal Medicine Residency Program

**Specialty:** Internal Medicine
**Program name:** Mount Carmel Health System Program
**Program code:** 140-38-12-341

**State:** Ohio
**Address:** Mount Carmel Health System, Department of Internal Medicine,
        793 W State St, Columbus, OH  43222
**Phone:** (614) 234-1079
**Fax:** (614) 234-1079
**Percentage of IMGs in the program:** 80%
**Minimum USMLE Step 1 Score Requirement:** No limits set
**Minimum USMLE Step 2 Score Requirement:** No limits set
**Attempts on any step:** Must pass on first attempt
**CS required at time of application:** No
**USCE Requirement:** Yes, 12 months
**Cut-Off time since graduation:** 5 years
**Program offers couple match:** Yes
**Visas Sponsored or accepted:** No visa

## Mercy St Vincent Medical Center/Mercy Health Partners Internal Medicine Residency Program

**Specialty:** Internal Medicine
**Program name:** Mercy St Vincent Medical Center/Mercy Health Partners Program
**Program code:** 140-38-12-533
**NRMP Code:** 1580140C0
**Program type:** Community-based university

affiliated hospital
**State:** Ohio
**Address:** Mercy St Vincent Medical Center,
2213 Cherry St, Toledo, OH  43608
**Phone:** (419) 251-4554
**Fax:** (419) 251-6795
**Percentage of IMGs in the program:** 100%
**Minimum USMLE Step 1 Score Requirement:**
No limits set
**Minimum USMLE Step 2 Score Requirement:**
No limits set
**Attempts on any step:** No limits set
**CS required at time of application:** Yes
including ECFMG certificate
**USCE Requirement:** None
**Cut-Off time since graduation:** No limits set but
prefer less than 5 years candidates
**Program offers couple match:** No
**Visas Sponsored or accepted:** J1 visa (and H1b
visa for select cases)


## Canton Medical Education Foundation/NEOMED Internal Medicine Residency Program

**Specialty:** Internal Medicine
**Program name:** Canton Medical Education
Foundation/NEOMED Program
**Program code:** 140-38-21-330
**NRMP Code:** 2009140C0

**Program type:** Community-based university affiliated hospital
**State:** Ohio
**Address:** Aultman Hospital, Internal Medicine Program,
2600 Sixth St SW, Canton, OH  44710
**Phone:** (330) 363-6220
**Fax:** (330) 588-2605
**Percentage of IMGs in the program:** 80%
**Minimum USMLE Step 1 Score Requirement:** No limits set
**Minimum USMLE Step 2 Score Requirement:** No limits set
**Attempts on any step:** No limits set
**CS required at time of application:** Yes including ECFMG certificate
**USCE Requirement:** None
**Cut-Off time since graduation:** 4 years
**Program offers couple match:** Yes
**Visas Sponsored or accepted:** J1 visa and H1b visa

## University of Cincinnati Medical Center/College of Medicine Internal Medicine Residency Program

**Specialty:** Internal Medicine
**Program name:** University of Cincinnati Medical Center/College of Medicine Program
**Program code:** 140-38-21-334

**NRMP Code:** 1548140C0, 1548140C1, 1548140P0
**Program type:** University-based
**State:** Ohio
**Address:** University Hospital University of Cincinnati,
          231 Albert Sabin Way, Cincinnati, OH 45267-0557
**Phone:** (513) 558-5235
**Fax:** (513) 558-3878
**Percentage of IMGs in the program:** 20%
**Minimum USMLE Step 1 Score Requirement:** 205
**Minimum USMLE Step 2 Score Requirement:** 205
**Attempts on any step:** No limits set
**CS required at time of application:** Yes including ECFMG certificate
**USCE Requirement:** Yes 2 months
**Cut-Off time since graduation:** 4 years
**Program offers couple match:** Yes
**Visas Sponsored or accepted:** J1 visa and H1b visa

## Case Western Reserve University/University Hospitals Case Medical Center Internal Medicine Residency Program

**Specialty:** Internal Medicine
**Program name:** Case Western Reserve University/University Hospitals Case Medical Center Program
**Program code:** 140-38-21-335
**Program type:** University-based
**State:** Ohio
**Address:** University Hospitals Case Medical Center,
          11100 Euclid Ave, Cleveland, OH 44106
**Phone:** (216) 844-5082
**Fax:** (216) 844-8216
**Percentage of IMGs in the program:** 10%
**Minimum USMLE Step 1 Score Requirement:** 210
**Minimum USMLE Step 2 Score Requirement:** 210
**Attempts on any step:** Must pass on first attempt
**CS required at time of application:** Yes including ECFMG certificate
**USCE Requirement:** None
**Cut-Off time since graduation:** 5 years
**Program offers couple match:** Yes
**Visas Sponsored or accepted:** J1 visa


## Fairview Hospital Internal Medicine Residency Program

**Specialty:** Internal Medicine
**Program name:** Fairview Hospital Program
**Program code:** 140-38-21-340
**NRMP Code:** 3187140P0, 3187140C0
**Program type:** Community-based
**State:** Ohio
**Address:** Fairview Hospital, 18101 Lorain Ave, Cleveland, OH  44111-5656
**Phone:** (216) 476-7029
**Fax:** (216) 476-2944
**Percentage of IMGs in the program:** 100%
**Minimum USMLE Step 1 Score Requirement:** 215
**Minimum USMLE Step 2 Score Requirement:** 215
**Attempts on any step:** Must pass on the first attempt including CS exam
**CS required at time of application:** Yes
**USCE Requirement:** None
**Cut-Off time since graduation:** 10 years
**Program offers couple match:** Yes
**Visas Sponsored or accepted:** J1 visa and H1b visa


## Wright State University Internal Medicine Residency Program

**Specialty:** Internal Medicine
**Program name:** Wright State University Program

**Program code:** 140-38-21-345
**NRMP Code:** 2011140C0
**Program type:** Community-based university affiliated hospital
**State:** Ohio
**Address:** Wright State University, Department of Internal Medicine 2nd Floor,
128 E Apple St, Dayton, OH  45409
**Phone:** (937) 208-2866
**Fax:** (937) 208-5304
**Percentage of IMGs in the program:** 20% (Varies)
**Minimum USMLE Step 1 Score Requirement:** 210
**Minimum USMLE Step 2 Score Requirement:** 210
**Attempts on any step:** Must pass on first attempt including CS exam
**CS required at time of application:** Yes including ECFMG certificate
**USCE Requirement:** Yes 2 months
**Cut-Off time since graduation:** 5 years
**Program offers couple match:** Yes
**Visas Sponsored or accepted:** No visa

## Kettering Medical Center Internal Medicine Residency Program

**Specialty:** Internal Medicine
**Program name:** Kettering Medical Center

Program
**Program code:** 140-38-21-347
**NRMP Code:** 1576140C0
**Program type:** Community-based university affiliated hospital
**State:** Ohio
**Address:** Kettering Medical Center, 3535 Southern Blvd, Kettering, OH  45429
**Phone:** (937) 395-8693
**Fax:** (937) 395-8399
**Percentage of IMGs in the program:** 20%
**Minimum USMLE Step 1 Score Requirement:** 205
**Minimum USMLE Step 2 Score Requirement:** 205
**Attempts on any step:** No limits set
**CS required at time of application:** No
**USCE Requirement:** None
**Cut-Off time since graduation:** 5 years
**Program offers couple match:** Yes
**Visas Sponsored or accepted:** J1 visa

## University of Toledo Internal Medicine Residency Program

**Specialty:** Internal Medicine
**Program name:** University of Toledo Program
**Program code:** 140-38-21-348
**NRMP Code:** 1579140P0, 1579140C0
**Program type:** University-based

**State:** Ohio
**Address:** University of Toledo Medical Center, 3000 Arlingtlon Ave, Toledo, OH  43614
**Phone:** (419) 383-6387
**Fax:** (419) 383-6180
**Percentage of IMGs in the program:** 30%
**Minimum USMLE Step 1 Score Requirement:** 212
**Minimum USMLE Step 2 Score Requirement:** 212
**Attempts on any step:** Must pass on first attempt including CS exam
**CS required at time of application:** Yes including ECFMG certificate
**USCE Requirement:** None
**Cut-Off time since graduation:** 5 years
**Program offers couple match:** Yes
**Visas Sponsored or accepted:** J1 visa

## TriHealth (Good Samaritan Hospital) Internal Medicine Residency Program

**Specialty:** Internal Medicine
**Program name:** TriHealth (Good Samaritan Hospital) Program
**Program code:** 140-38-31-332
**NRMP Code:** 1550140P0, 1550140C0
**Program type:** Community-based university affiliated hospital

**State:** Ohio
**Address:** Good Samaritan Hospital, Department of Medicine,
375 Dixmyth Ave, Cincinnati, OH 45220-2489
**Phone:** (513) 862-3229
**Fax:** (513) 221-5865
**Percentage of IMGs in the program:** 60%
**Minimum USMLE Step 1 Score Requirement:** No limits set
**Minimum USMLE Step 2 Score Requirement:** No limits set
**Attempts on any step:** No limits set
**CS required at time of application:** Yes including ECFMG certificate
**USCE Requirement:** None
**Cut-Off time since graduation:** 5 years
**Program offers couple match:** No
**Visas Sponsored or accepted:** J1 visa and H1b visa

# Western Reserve Health Education/NEOMED Internal Medicine Residency Program

**Specialty:** Internal Medicine
**Program name:** Western Reserve Health Education/NEOMED Program
**Program code:** 140-38-31-350
**NRMP Code:** 1585140C0, 1585140P0

**Program type:** Community-based university affiliated hospital
**State:** Ohio
**Address:** Western Reserve Health Education Inc,

      500 Gypsy Ln, Youngstown, OH 44501-0990
**Phone:** (330) 884-5812
**Fax:** (330) 884-5688
**Percentage of IMGs in the program:** 90%
**Minimum USMLE Step 1 Score Requirement:** 220
**Minimum USMLE Step 2 Score Requirement:** 220
**Attempts on any step:** Must pass on first attempt
**CS required at time of application:** Yes including ECFMG certificate
**USCE Requirement:** None
**Cut-Off time since graduation:** No limits set
**Program offers couple match:** Yes
**Visas Sponsored or accepted:** J1 visa


## Oklahoma


## University of Oklahoma Health Sciences Center Internal Medicine Residency Program

**Specialty:** Internal Medicine
**Program name:** University of Oklahoma Health Sciences Center Program
**Program code:** 140-39-21-351
**NRMP Code:** 1588140P0, 1588140C0
**Program type:** University-based
**State:** Oklahoma
**Address:** University of Oklahoma Health Sciences Center,
          920 Stanton L Young Blvd, Oklahoma City, OK  73126-0901
**Phone:** (405) 271-5963
**Fax:** (405) 271-7186
**Percentage of IMGs in the program:** 30%
**Minimum USMLE Step 1 Score Requirement:** 205
**Minimum USMLE Step 2 Score Requirement:** 205
**Attempts on any step:** Must pass on first attempt
**CS required at time of application:** No
**USCE Requirement:** None
**Cut-Off time since graduation:** 5 years
**Program offers couple match:** Yes
**Visas Sponsored or accepted:** J1 visa

## University of Oklahoma College of Medicine-Tulsa Internal Medicine Residency Program

**Specialty:** Internal Medicine
**Program name:** University of Oklahoma College of Medicine-Tulsa Program
**Program code:** 140-39-21-352
**NRMP Code:** 2727140P0, 2727140C0
**Program type:** University-based
**State:** Oklahoma
**Address:** University of Oklahoma College of Medicine-Tulsa,

> Department of Internal Medicine,
> 4502 E 41st St, Tulsa, OK  74135

**Phone:** (918) 660-3428
**Percentage of IMGs in the program:** 50%
**Minimum USMLE Step 1 Score Requirement:** 205
**Minimum USMLE Step 2 Score Requirement:** 205
**Attempts on any step:** Must pass maximum on 2nd attempt
**CS required at time of application:** Yes
**USCE Requirement:** Yes, 3 months
**Cut-Off time since graduation:** No limits set
**Program offers couple match:** Yes
**Visas Sponsored or accepted:** J1 visa (and H1b visa for exceptional candidates)

# Oregon

## Legacy Emanuel Hospital and Health Center Internal Medicine Residency Program

**Specialty:** Internal Medicine
**Program name:** Legacy Emanuel Hospital and Health Center Program
**Program code:** 140-40-11-353
**NRMP Code:** 1594140C0
**Program type:** Community-based university affiliated hospital
**State:** Oregon
**Address:** Legacy Good Samaritan Medical Center,
        1015 NW 22nd Ave, Portland, OR 97210
**Phone:** (503) 413-7036
**Fax:** (503) 413-7361
**Percentage of IMGs in the program:** 10%
**Minimum USMLE Step 1 Score Requirement:** No limits set
**Minimum USMLE Step 2 Score Requirement:** No limits set
**Attempts on any step:** No limits set

**CS required at time of application:** No
**USCE Requirement:** Yes, at least 1 month but 3 months preferred
**Cut-Off time since graduation:** 5 years
**Program offers couple match:** Yes
**Visas Sponsored or accepted:** J1 visa and H1b visa

## Providence Health & Services-Oregon/St Vincent Hospital and Medical Center Internal Medicine Residency Program

**Specialty:** Internal Medicine
**Program name:** Providence Health & Services-Oregon/St Vincent Hospital and Medical Center Program
**Program code:** 140-40-31-356
**NRMP Code:** 1598140P0, 1598140C0
**Program type:** Community-based university affiliated hospital
**State:** Oregon
**Address:** St Vincent Hospital and Medical Center, Suite 20,
        9205 SW Barnes Rd, Portland, OR 97225
**Phone:** (503) 216-2401
**Fax:** (503) 216-4041
**Percentage of IMGs in the program:** 15%

**Minimum USMLE Step 1 Score Requirement:**
No limits set
**Minimum USMLE Step 2 Score Requirement:**
No limits set
**Attempts on any step:** No limits set
**CS required at time of application:** No
**USCE Requirement:** None
**Cut-Off time since graduation:** 5 years
**Program offers couple match:** Yes
**Visas Sponsored or accepted:** No visa

## Oregon Health & Science University Internal Medicine Residency Program

**Specialty:** Internal Medicine
**Program name:** Oregon Health & Science University Program
**Program code:** 140-40-31-357
**NRMP Code:** 1599140C0
**Program type:** University-based
**State:** Oregon
**Address:** Oregon Health & Science University, Department of Medicine OP-30,
          3181 SW Sam Jackson Park Rd, Portland, OR  97239-3098
**Phone:** (503) 494-8530
**Fax:** (503) 494-5636
**Percentage of IMGs in the program:** 5%
**Minimum USMLE Step 1 Score Requirement:**

No limits set but prefer >230
**Minimum USMLE Step 2 Score Requirement:**
No limits set but prefer >230
**Attempts on any step:** No limits set but prefer passing on first attempt
**CS required at time of application:** Yes
**USCE Requirement:** Yes, 1 year
**Cut-Off time since graduation:** 5 years
**Program offers couple match:** Yes
**Visas Sponsored or accepted:** J1 visa and H1b visa

## Pennsylvania

### Geisinger Health System Internal Medicine Residency Program

**Specialty:** Internal Medicine
**Program name:** Geisinger Health System Program
**Program code:** 140-41-11-362
**NRMP Code:** 1608140C0, 1608140P0
**Program type:** Community-based university affiliated hospital
**State:** Pennsylvania
**Address:** Geisinger Medical Center, Department of Medicine,
            100 N Academy Ave, Danville, PA

17822
**Phone:** (570) 271-6787
**Fax:** (570) 271-5734
**Percentage of IMGs in the program:** 50%
**Minimum USMLE Step 1 Score Requirement:**
205
**Minimum USMLE Step 2 Score Requirement:**
205
**Attempts on any step:** Must pass on first
attempt
**CS required at time of application:** No
**USCE Requirement:** None
**Cut-Off time since graduation:** 10 years
**Program offers couple match:** Yes
**Visas Sponsored or accepted:** J1 visa and H1b
visa

## Easton Hospital Internal Medicine Residency Program

**Specialty:** Internal Medicine
**Program name:** Easton Hospital Program
**Program code:** 140-41-11-363
**Program type:** Community-based university
affiliated hospital
**State:** Pennsylvania
**Address:** Easton Hospital, Meuser Building,
          250 S 21st St, Easton, PA  18042-3892
**Phone:** (610) 250-4517

**Fax:** (610) 250-4833
**Percentage of IMGs in the program:** 60%
**Minimum USMLE Step 1 Score Requirement:** 220
**Minimum USMLE Step 2 Score Requirement:** 220
**Attempts on any step:** Must pass on first attempt
**CS required at time of application:** Yes
**USCE Requirement:** None
**Cut-Off time since graduation:** 5 years
**Program offers couple match:** No
**Visas Sponsored or accepted:** No visa

## PinnacleHealth Hospitals Internal Medicine Residency Program

**Specialty:** Internal Medicine
**Program name:** PinnacleHealth Hospitals Program
**Program code:** 140-41-11-365
**State:** Pennsylvania
**Address:** Pinnacle Health Hospitals, Department of Medicine,
         PO Box 8700, Harrisburg, PA  17105-9011
**Phone:** (717) 231-8506
**Fax:** (717) 231-8535
**Percentage of IMGs in the program:** 50%

**Minimum USMLE Step 1 Score Requirement:** 210

**Minimum USMLE Step 2 Score Requirement:** 210

**Attempts on any step:** Must pass on first attempt

**CS required at time of application:** No

**USCE Requirement:** Yes 1 month

**Cut-Off time since graduation:** 5 years

**Program offers couple match:** Yes

**Visas Sponsored or accepted:** J1 visa and H1b visa

## Penn State Milton S Hershey Medical Center Internal Medicine Residency Program

**Specialty:** Internal Medicine

**Program name:** Penn State Milton S Hershey Medical Center Program

**Program code:** 140-41-11-366

**State:** Pennsylvania

**Address:** Penn State Milton S Hershey Medical Center,

PO Box 850 Department of Medicine H039

500 University Dr, Hershey, PA 17033

**Phone:** (717) 531-8390

**Fax:** (717) 531-5831

**Percentage of IMGs in the program:** 50%

**Minimum USMLE Step 1 Score Requirement:**
No limits set but prefer above 210
**Minimum USMLE Step 2 Score Requirement:**
No limits set but prefer above 210
**Attempts on any step:** No limits set
**CS required at time of application:** Yes
**USCE Requirement:** No but 1 year is preferred
**Cut-Off time since graduation:** 5 years
**Program offers couple match:** Yes
**Visas Sponsored or accepted:** J1 visa

## Albert Einstein Healthcare Network Internal Medicine Residency Program

**Specialty:** Internal Medicine
**Program name:** Albert Einstein Healthcare
Network Program
**Program code:** 140-41-11-369
**NRMP Code:** 1631140P0, 1631140C0,
1631140P1
**Program type:** Community-based university
affiliated hospital
**State:** Pennsylvania
**Address:** Albert Einstein Medical Center,
Department of Medicine Suite 363,
        5401 Old York Road, Philadelphia, PA
19141-3025
**Phone**: (800) 220-2362

**Fax:** (215) 456-7926
**Percentage of IMGs in the program:** 30%
**Minimum USMLE Step 1 Score Requirement:**
No limits set
**Minimum USMLE Step 2 Score Requirement:**
No limits set
**Attempts on any step:** No limits set
**CS required at time of application:** Yes
**USCE Requirement:** None
**Cut-Off time since graduation:** No limits set
**Program offers couple match:** Yes
**Visas Sponsored or accepted:** J1 visa and H1b
visa

## Lankenau Medical Center Internal Medicine Residency Program

**Specialty:** Internal Medicine
**Program name:** Lankenau Medical Center
Program
**Program code:** 140-41-11-373
**NRMP Code:** 1632140P0, 1632140C0
**Program type:** Community-based university
affiliated hospital
**State:** Pennsylvania
**Address:** Lankenau Medical Center, Annenberg
Conference Center Suite G10,
          100 Lancaster Ave, Wynnewood, PA
19096
**Phone:** (484) 476-6840

**Fax:** (484) 476-8141
**Percentage of IMGs in the program:** 20%
**Minimum USMLE Step 1 Score Requirement:** No limits set
**Minimum USMLE Step 2 Score Requirement:** No limits set
**Attempts on any step:** Must pass on first attempt
**CS required at time of application:** No
**USCE Requirement:** None
**Cut-Off time since graduation:** 5 years
**Program offers couple match:** Yes
**Visas Sponsored or accepted:** J1 visa and H1b visa

## Mercy Catholic Medical Center Internal Medicine Residency Program

**Specialty:** Internal Medicine
**Program name:** Mercy Catholic Medical Center Program
**Program code:** 140-41-11-375
**NRMP Code:** 1636140P0, 1636140P1, 1636140C0
**Program type:** Community-based university affiliated hospital
**State:** Pennsylvania
**Address:** Mercy Catholic Medical Center, 1500 Lansdowne Ave, Darby, PA

19023
**Phone:** (610) 237 4958
**Percentage of IMGs in the program:** 50%
**Minimum USMLE Step 1 Score Requirement:**
No limits set
**Minimum USMLE Step 2 Score Requirement:**
No limits set
**Attempts on any step:** No limits set
**CS required at time of application:** Yes
including ECFMG certificate
**USCE Requirement:** Yes, 1 month
**Cut-Off time since graduation:** No limits set
**Program offers couple match:** Yes
**Visas Sponsored or accepted:** J1 visa and H1b
visa

## Pennsylvania Hospital of the University of Pennsylvania Health System Internal Medicine Residency Program

**Specialty:** Internal Medicine
**Program name:** Pennsylvania Hospital of the
University of Pennsylvania Health System
Program
**Program code:** 140-41-11-376
**NRMP Code:**
**Program type:**
**State:** Pennsylvania
**Address:** Pennsylvania Hospital, Department of

Medicine 1 Pine West,
            800 Spruce Street, Philadelphia, PA
19107
**Phone:** (215) 829-5410
**Fax:** (215) 829-7129
**Percentage of IMGs in the program:** 30%
**Minimum USMLE Step 1 Score Requirement:**
No limits set
**Minimum USMLE Step 2 Score Requirement:**
No limits set
**Attempts on any step:** Must pass on first
attempt
**CS required at time of application:** No
**USCE Requirement:** None
**Cut-Off time since graduation:** No limits set
**Program offers couple match:** No
**Visas Sponsored or accepted:** J1 visa and H1b
visa

# Allegheny General Hospital-Western Pennsylvania Hospital Medical Education Consortium (AGH) Internal Medicine Residency Program

**Specialty:** Internal Medicine
**Program name:** Allegheny General Hospital-Western Pennsylvania Hospital Medical Education Consortium (AGH) Program

**Program code:** 140-41-11-381
**NRMP Code:** 1648140C0, 1648140P0, 1648140P1, 1648140C1
**Program type:** Community-based university affiliated hospital
**State:** Pennsylvania
**Address:** Allegheny General Hospital, Department of Internal Medicine,
320 E North Ave, Pittsburgh, PA 15212-9986
**Phone:** (412) 359-4970
**Fax:** (412) 359-4983
**Percentage of IMGs in the program:** 60%
**Minimum USMLE Step 1 Score Requirement:** 220
**Minimum USMLE Step 2 Score Requirement:** 220
**Attempts on any step:** Must pass maximum on the 2nd attempt on any step
**CS required at time of application:** Yes
**USCE Requirement:** Yes, 1-2 months with 1-2 US LORs
**Cut-Off time since graduation:** No limits set
**Program offers couple match:** Yes
**Visas Sponsored or accepted:** J1 visa

## UPMC Medical Education (Mercy) Internal Medicine Residency Program

**Specialty:** Internal Medicine
**Program name:** UPMC Medical Education (Mercy) Program
**Program code:** 140-41-11-385
**NRMP Code:** 1649140C0
**Program type:** Community-based university affiliated hospital
**State:** Pennsylvania
**Address:** UPMC Mercy, Department of Medicine,
          1400 Locust St, Pittsburgh, PA 15219-5166
**Phone:** (800) 637-2946
**Fax:** (412) 232-5689
**Percentage of IMGs in the program:** 40%
**Minimum USMLE Step 1 Score Requirement:** 220
**Minimum USMLE Step 2 Score Requirement:** 220
**Attempts on any step:** Must pass on first attempt
**CS required at time of application:** No
**USCE Requirement:** Yes 1-2 months
**Cut-Off time since graduation:** 6 years
**Program offers couple match:** Yes
**Visas Sponsored or accepted:** J1 visa

## York Hospital Internal Medicine Residency Program

**Specialty:** Internal Medicine
**Program name:** York Hospital Program
**Program code:** 140-41-11-392
**NRMP Code:** 1674140C0
**Program type:** Community-based university affiliated hospital
**State:** Pennsylvania
**Address:** York Hospital, Department of Internal Medicine,
           1001 S George St, York, PA  17405
**Phone:** (717) 851-2164
**Fax:** (717) 851-2843
**Percentage of IMGs in the program:** 50%
**Minimum USMLE Step 1 Score Requirement:** No limits set
**Minimum USMLE Step 2 Score Requirement:** No limits set
**Attempts on any step:** Must pass on first attempt
**CS required at time of application:** No
**USCE Requirement:** None
**Cut-Off time since graduation:** No limits set
**Program offers couple match:** Yes
**Visas Sponsored or accepted:** J1 visa and H1b visa

# Abington Memorial Hospital Internal Medicine Residency Program

**Specialty:** Internal Medicine
**Program name:** Abington Memorial Hospital Program
**Program code:** 140-41-12-358
**NRMP Code:** 1600140P0
**Program type:** Community-based university affiliated hospital
**State:** Pennsylvania
**Address:** Abington Memorial Hospital, Elkins 2B, 1200 Old York Rd, Abington, PA  19001
**Phone:** (215) 481-2056
**Fax:** (215) 481-4361
**Percentage of IMGs in the program:** 50%
**Minimum USMLE Step 1 Score Requirement:** 217
**Minimum USMLE Step 2 Score Requirement:** 217
**Attempts on any step:** Must pass on first attempt
**CS required at time of application:** Yes
**USCE Requirement:** None
**Cut-Off time since graduation:** 5 years
**Program offers couple match:** No
**Visas Sponsored or accepted:** J1 visa and H1b visa

# Robert Packer Hospital/Guthrie Internal Medicine Residency Program

**Specialty:** Internal Medicine
**Program name:** Robert Packer Hospital/Guthrie Program
**Program code:** 140-41-12-389
**NRMP Code:** 1664140C0
**Program type:** Community-based university affiliated hospital
**State:** Pennsylvania
**Address:** Guthrie/Robert Packer Hospital, Internal Medicine Program,
          One Guthrie Sq, Sayre, PA  18840-1698
**Phone:** (570) 887-4559
**Fax:** (570) 887-5352
**Percentage of IMGs in the program:** 50%
**Minimum USMLE Step 1 Score Requirement:** 205
**Minimum USMLE Step 2 Score Requirement:** 205
**Attempts on any step:** No limits set
**CS required at time of application:** Yes including ECFMG certificate
**USCE Requirement:** None
**Cut-Off time since graduation:** No limits set
**Program offers couple match:** Yes
**Visas Sponsored or accepted:** J1 visa and H1b visa

# UPMC Medical Education (McKeesport Hospital) Internal Medicine Residency Program

**Specialty:** Internal Medicine
**Program name:** UPMC Medical Education (McKeesport Hospital) Program
**Program code:** 140-41-21-368
**NRMP Code:** 1620140C0
**Program type:** Community-based university affiliated hospital
**State:** Pennsylvania
**Address:** UPMC McKeesport Hospital, Department of Medicine,
          1500 Fifth Ave, McKeesport, PA 15132
**Phone:** (412) 664-2167
**Fax:** (412) 664-2164
**Percentage of IMGs in the program:** 80%
**Minimum USMLE Step 1 Score Requirement:** 215
**Minimum USMLE Step 2 Score Requirement:** 215
**Attempts on any step:** Must pass on first attempt
**CS required at time of application:** Yes including ECFMG certificate
**USCE Requirement:** None
**Cut-Off time since graduation:** 3 years
**Program offers couple match:** Yes

**Visas Sponsored or accepted:** J1 visa and H1b visa

## Drexel University College of Medicine/Hahnemann University Hospital Internal Medicine Residency Program

**Specialty:** Internal Medicine
**Program name:** Drexel University College of Medicine/Hahnemann University Hospital Program
**Program code:** 140-41-21-374
**NRMP Code:** 1849140P0, 1849140C0
**Program type:** University-based
**State:** Pennsylvania
**Address:** Hahnemann University Hospital, 245 N 15th St, Philadelphia, PA 19102
**Phone:** (215) 762-7916
**Fax:** (215) 762-7765
**Percentage of IMGs in the program:** 30%
**Minimum USMLE Step 1 Score Requirement:** No limits set
**Minimum USMLE Step 2 Score Requirement:** No limits set
**Attempts on any step:** Must pass on first attempt
**CS required at time of application:** No
**USCE Requirement:** None but 1 month preferred

**Cut-Off time since graduation:** No limits set
**Program offers couple match:** Yes
**Visas Sponsored or accepted:** J1 visa

## Temple University Hospital Internal Medicine Residency Program

**Specialty:** Internal Medicine
**Program name:** Temple University Hospital Program
**Program code:** 140-41-21-378
**NRMP Code:** 1646140C0, 1646140P0
**Program type:** University-based
**State:** Pennsylvania
**Address:** Temple University Hospital, Department of Medicine,
3401 N Broad St, Philadelphia, PA 19140
**Phone**: (215) 707-5734
**Fax:** (215) 707-5978
**Percentage of IMGs in the program:** 5%
**Minimum USMLE Step 1 Score Requirement:** 220
**Minimum USMLE Step 2 Score Requirement:** 220
**Attempts on any step:** No limits set
**CS required at time of application:** No
**USCE Requirement:** Yes, 1 month
**Cut-Off time since graduation:** No limits set
**Program offers couple match:** Yes

**Visas Sponsored or accepted:** J1 visa and H1b visa

## Reading Health System Internal Medicine Residency Program

**Specialty:** Internal Medicine
**Program name:** Reading Health System Program
**Program code:** 140-41-21-388
**NRMP Code:** 1661140C0
**Program type:** Community-based university affiliated hospital
**State:** Pennsylvania
**Address:** Reading Hospital, Department of Medicine,
            Sixth Ave & Spruce Streets, West Reading, PA  19611
**Phone:** (484) 628-8133
**Fax:** (484) 628-9003
**Percentage of IMGs in the program:** 40%
**Minimum USMLE Step 1 Score Requirement:** 205
**Minimum USMLE Step 2 Score Requirement:** 205
**Attempts on any step:** No limits set
**CS required at time of application:** No
**USCE Requirement:** None
**Cut-Off time since graduation:** No limits set

**Program offers couple match:** Yes
**Visas Sponsored or accepted:** J1 visa and H1b visa

## Wright Center for Graduate Medical Education Internal Medicine Residency Program

**Specialty:** Internal Medicine
**Program name:** Wright Center for Graduate Medical Education Program
**Program code:** 140-41-21-390
**Program type:** Community-based
**State:** Pennsylvania
**Address:** Wright Center for Graduate Med Education, Department of Medicine,
      501 Madison Ave, Scranton, PA  18510
**Phone:** (570) 343-2383
**Fax:** (570) 343-4800
**Percentage of IMGs in the program:** 80%
**Minimum USMLE Step 1 Score Requirement:** 205
**Minimum USMLE Step 2 Score Requirement:** 205
**Attempts on any step:** No limits set
**CS required at time of application:** No
**USCE Requirement:** None
**Cut-Off time since graduation:** No limits set
**Program offers couple match:** Yes

**Visas Sponsored or accepted:** J1 visa and H1b visa

## UPMC Medical Education Internal Medicine Residency Program

**Specialty:** Internal Medicine
**Program name:** UPMC Medical Education Program
**Program code:** 140-41-21-504
**NRMP Code:** 1652140C1, 1652140C0, 1657140C0, 1652140P0
**Program type:** University-based
**State:** Pennsylvania
**Address:** University of Pittsburgh Medical Center
     200 Lothrop St, Pittsburgh, PA  15213
**Phone:** (412) 692-4942
**Fax:** (412) 692-4944
**Percentage of IMGs in the program:** 20%
**Minimum USMLE Step 1 Score Requirement:** 225
**Minimum USMLE Step 2 Score Requirement:** 225
**Attempts on any step:** No limits set
**CS required at time of application:** No
**USCE Requirement:** None
**Cut-Off time since graduation:** 5 years
**Program offers couple match:** Yes
**Visas Sponsored or accepted:** J1 visa

# St Luke's Hospital Internal Medicine Residency Program

**Specialty:** Internal Medicine
**Program name:** St Luke's Hospital Program
**Program code:** 140-41-31-360
**NRMP Code:** University-based
**Program type:** 1605140C0
**State:** Pennsylvania
**Address:** St Luke's University Hospital, Department of Medicine,
       801 Ostrum St, Bethlehem, PA  18015
**Phone:** (484) 526-4644
**Fax:** (484) 526-4920
**Percentage of IMGs in the program:** 40%
**Minimum USMLE Step 1 Score Requirement:** No limits set
**Minimum USMLE Step 2 Score Requirement:** No limits set
**Attempts on any step:** No limits set but prefer pass on first attempt
**CS required at time of application:** Yes including ECFMG certificate
**USCE Requirement:** None but prefer 1-2 months of observerships
**Cut-Off time since graduation:** No limits set
**Program offers couple match:** Yes
**Visas Sponsored or accepted:** J1 visa and H1b visa

# Conemaugh Valley Memorial Hospital Internal Medicine Residency Program

**Specialty:** Internal Medicine
**Program name:** Conemaugh Valley Memorial Hospital Program
**Program code:** 140-41-31-367
**NRMP Code:** 1616140P0, 1616140C0
**Program type:** Community-based university affiliated hospital
**State:** Pennsylvania
**Address:** Conemaugh Memorial Medical Center, Department of Medicine,
          1086 Franklin St, Johnstown, PA 15905
**Phone:** (814) 534-9408
**Fax:** (814) 534-3290
**Percentage of IMGs in the program:** 100%
**Minimum USMLE Step 1 Score Requirement:** No limits set
**Minimum USMLE Step 2 Score Requirement:** No limits set
**Attempts on any step:** No limits set
**CS required at time of application:** Yes including ECFMG certificate
**USCE Requirement:** Yes, 2 months
**Cut-Off time since graduation:** 5 years
**Program offers couple match:** Yes

**Visas Sponsored or accepted:** J1 visa and H1b visa

## Crozer-Chester Medical Center Internal Medicine Residency Program

**Specialty:** Internal Medicine
**Program name:** Crozer-Chester Medical Center Program
**Program code:** 140-41-31-514
**NRMP Code:** 3185140C0
**Program type:** Community-based university affiliated hospital
**State:** Pennsylvania
**Address:** Crozer-Chester Medical Center,
        Department of Medicine 3rd Floor East Wing,
        One Medical Center Blvd, Upland, PA 19013
**Phone:** (610) 874-6114
**Fax:** (610) 447-6373
**Percentage of IMGs in the program:** 70%
**Minimum USMLE Step 1 Score Requirement:** No limits set
**Minimum USMLE Step 2 Score Requirement:** No limits set
**Attempts on any step:** Must pass on first attempt
**CS required at time of application:** Yes

including ECFMG certificate
**USCE Requirement:** None
**Cut-Off time since graduation:** 4 years
**Program offers couple match:** Yes
**Visas Sponsored or accepted:** J1 visa

# Rhode Island

## Memorial Hospital of Rhode Island/Brown University Internal Medicine Residency Program

**Specialty:** Internal Medicine
**Program name:** Memorial Hospital of Rhode Island/Brown University Program
**Program code:** 140-43-21-473
**NRMP Code:** 1676140M0
**Program type:** Community-based university affiliated hospital
**State:** Rhode Island
**Address:** Memorial Hospital Rhode Island, Department of Medicine,
          111 Brewster St, Pawtucket, RI  02860
**Phone:** (401) 729-2221
**Fax:** (401) 729-2202
**Percentage of IMGs in the program:** 100%

**Minimum USMLE Step 1 Score Requirement:** 220
**Minimum USMLE Step 2 Score Requirement:** 220
**Attempts on any step:** Must pass maximum on the 2nd attempt
**CS required at time of application:** No
**USCE Requirement:** None
**Cut-Off time since graduation:** No limits set
**Program offers couple match:** Yes
**Visas Sponsored or accepted:** J1 visa and H1b visa

## Roger Williams Medical Center Internal Medicine Residency Program

**Specialty:** Internal Medicine
**Program name:** Roger Williams Medical Center Program
**Program code:** 140-43-31-401
**NRMP Code:** 1678140C0, 1678140P0
**Program type:** Community-based university affiliated hospital
**State:** Rhode Island
**Address:** Roger Williams Medical Center, Department of Medicine,
825 Chalkstone Ave, Providence, RI 02908
**Phone:** (401) 456-2393

**Fax:** (401) 456-6809
**Percentage of IMGs in the program:** 50%
**Minimum USMLE Step 1 Score Requirement:** 210
**Minimum USMLE Step 2 Score Requirement:** 210
**Attempts on any step:** Must pass on first attempt
**CS required at time of application:** No
**USCE Requirement:** 1year
**Cut-Off time since graduation:** 5 years
**Program offers couple match:** Yes
**Visas Sponsored or accepted:** J1 visa

# South Carolina

## Greenville Health System/University of South Carolina Internal Medicine Residency Program

**Specialty:** Internal Medicine
**Program name:** Greenville Health System/University of South Carolina Program
**Program code:** 140-45-11-405

**NRMP Code:** 1683140C0, 1683140P0
**Program type:** University-based
**State:** South Carolina
**Address:** Greenville Hospital System, Department of Internal Medicine,
     701 Grove Rd, Greenville, SC  29605
**Phone:** (864) 455-7882
**Fax:** (864) 455-5008
**Percentage of IMGs in the program:** 0%-10% variable from match to match
**Minimum USMLE Step 1 Score Requirement:** No limits set
**Minimum USMLE Step 2 Score Requirement:** No limits set
**Attempts on any step:** Must pass on the first attempt
**CS required at time of application:** Yes
**USCE Requirement:** 3 months
**Cut-Off time since graduation:** 3 years
**Program offers couple match:** Yes
**Visas Sponsored or accepted:** J1 visa

## Medical University of South Carolina Internal Medicine Residency Program

**Specialty:** Internal Medicine
**Program name:** Medical University of South Carolina Program
**Program code:** 140-45-21-403

**NRMP Code:** 1680140C0, 1680140P0
**Program type:** University-based
**State:** South Carolina
**Address:** Medical University of South Carolina,
96 Jonathan Lucas St, Charleston, SC 29425
**Phone:** (843) 792-2731
**Fax:** (843) 792-0448
**Percentage of IMGs in the program:** 5%
**Minimum USMLE Step 1 Score Requirement:** 220
**Minimum USMLE Step 2 Score Requirement:** 220
**Attempts on any step:** Must pass on first attempt
**CS required at time of application:** Yes including ECFMG certificate
**USCE Requirement:** 1 year
**Cut-Off time since graduation:** 2 years
**Program offers couple match:** Yes
**Visas Sponsored or accepted:** J1 visa

# South Dakota

## University of South Dakota Internal Medicine Residency Program

**Specialty:** Internal Medicine

**Program name:** University of South Dakota Program
**Program code:** 140-46-21-406
**NRMP Code:** 2805140C0, 2805140P0
**Program type:** Community-based university affiliated hospital
**State:** South Dakota
**Address:** USD Sanford School of Medicine, Department of Medicine,
  1400 W 22nd St, Sioux Falls, SD 57105-1570
**Phone:** (605) 357-1558
**Fax:** (605) 357-1365
**Percentage of IMGs in the program:** 50%
**Minimum USMLE Step 1 Score Requirement:** 220
**Minimum USMLE Step 2 Score Requirement:** 220
**Attempts on any step:** Must pass on first attempt including CS exam
**CS required at time of application:** Yes
**USCE Requirement:** Yes at least 2 month with 2 US LOR, 1 year preferred
**Cut-Off time since graduation:** 5 years strongly preferred and must be clinically active
**Program offers couple match:** Yes
**Visas Sponsored or accepted:** J1 visa and H1b visa

# Tennessee

## University of Tennessee College of Medicine at Chattanooga Internal Medicine Residency Program

**Specialty:** Internal Medicine
**Program name:** University of Tennessee College of Medicine at Chattanooga Program
**Program code:** 140-47-11-407
**NRMP Code:** 1689140C0
**Program type:** University-based
**State:** Tennessee
**Address:** University of Tennessee College of Medicine-Chattanooga,
Department of Medicine Box 94,
975 E Third St, Chattanooga, TN  37403
**Phone:** (423) 778-2998
**Fax:** (423) 778-2611
**Percentage of IMGs in the program:** 60%
**Minimum USMLE Step 1 Score Requirement:** 210
**Minimum USMLE Step 2 Score Requirement:** 210
**Attempts on any step:** No limits set
**CS required at time of application:** No
**USCE Requirement:** None
**Cut-Off time since graduation:** No limits set
**Program offers couple match:** Yes
**Visas Sponsored or accepted:** J1 visa

# University of Tennessee Medical Center at Knoxville Internal Medicine Residency Program

**Specialty:** Internal Medicine
**Program name:** University of Tennessee Medical Center at Knoxville Program
**Program code:** 140-47-11-409
**NRMP Code:** 1839140C0
**Program type:** University-based
**State:** Tennessee
**Address:** University of Tennessee Memorial Hospital, Department of Medicine U-114,
            1924 Alcoa Hwy, Knoxville, TN  37920
**Phone:** (865) 305-9340    Ext:  6501
**Fax:** (865) 305-6849
**Percentage of IMGs in the program:** 10%
**Minimum USMLE Step 1 Score Requirement:** No limits set
**Minimum USMLE Step 2 Score Requirement:** No limits set
**Attempts on any step:** Must pass on first attempt
**CS required at time of application:** Yes including ECFMG certificate
**USCE Requirement:** Yes
**Cut-Off time since graduation:** 5 years unless clinically or research active
**Program offers couple match:** Yes
**Visas Sponsored or accepted:** J1 visa

## Meharry Medical College Internal Medicine Residency Program

**Specialty:** Internal Medicine
**Program name:** Meharry Medical College Program
**Program code:** 140-47-11-413
**NRMP Code:** 1028140C0
**Program type:** Community-based university affiliated hospital
**State:** Tennessee
**Address:** Meharry Medical College, Department of Internal Medicine,
1005 Dr D B Todd Jr Blvd, Nashville, TN 37208
**Phone:** (615) 327-6611
**Fax:** (615) 327-6733
**Percentage of IMGs in the program:** 50%
**Minimum USMLE Step 1 Score Requirement:** 215
**Minimum USMLE Step 2 Score Requirement:** 215
**Attempts on any step:** No limits set
**CS required at time of application:** Yes including ECFMG certificate
**USCE Requirement:** None
**Cut-Off time since graduation:** 5 years unless clinically or research active
**Program offers couple match:** Yes
**Visas Sponsored or accepted:** No visa

# East Tennessee State University Internal Medicine Residency Program

**Specialty:** Internal Medicine
**Program name:** East Tennessee State University Program
**Program code:** 140-47-21-408
**NRMP Code:** 2066140C0, 2066140P0
**Program type:** University-based
**State:** Tennessee
**Address:** ETSU James H Quillen College of Medicine, Internal Medicine Program,
        PO Box 70622, Johnson City, TN 37614
**Phone:** (423) 439-6286
**Percentage of IMGs in the program:** 50%
**Minimum USMLE Step 1 Score Requirement:** No limits set
**Minimum USMLE Step 2 Score Requirement:** No limits set
**Attempts on any step:** Total of one failed attempt allowed as sum in your final transcript
**CS required at time of application:** Yes including ECFMG certificate
**USCE Requirement:** None
**Cut-Off time since graduation:** 3 years, however if clinically active then 5 years
**Program offers couple match:** Yes
**Visas Sponsored or accepted:** J1 visa

# University of Tennessee Internal Medicine Residency Program

**Specialty:** Internal Medicine
**Program name:** University of Tennessee Program
**Program code:** 140-47-21-412
**NRMP Code:** 1844140P1, 1844140P0, 1844140C0, 1844140M0
**Program type:** University-based
**State:** Tennessee
**Address:** University of Tennessee Medical Center,
  Department of Medicine Room H314,
  956 Court Ave, Memphis, TN  38163
**Phone:** (901) 448-5704
**Fax:** (901) 448-7836
**Percentage of IMGs in the program:** 30%
**Minimum USMLE Step 1 Score Requirement:** No limits set
**Minimum USMLE Step 2 Score Requirement:** No limits set
**Attempts on any step:** Must pass on first attempt
**CS required at time of application:** No
**USCE Requirement:** None
**Cut-Off time since graduation:** 3 years, otherwise 5 years if clinically active
**Program offers couple match:** Yes
**Visas Sponsored or accepted:** J1 visa

# Texas

## University of Texas Health Science Center at Tyler/Good Shepherd Medical Center (Longview) Internal Medicine Residency Program

**Specialty:** Internal Medicine
**Program name:** University of Texas Health Science Center at Tyler/Good Shepherd Medical Center (Longview) Program
**Program code:** 140-48-00-890
**NRMP Code:** 3626140C0
**Program type:** Community-based university affiliated hospital
**State:** Texas
**Address:** Good Shepherd Medical Center, GME Office

    700 E Marshall Ave, Longview, TX 75601
**Phone:** (903) 315-5171
**Percentage of IMGs in the program:** 40%
**Minimum USMLE Step 1 Score Requirement:** No limits set but prefers 210
**Minimum USMLE Step 2 Score Requirement:** No limits set but prefers 210

**Attempts on any step:** No limits set
**CS required at time of application:** Yes
including ECFMG certificate
**USCE Requirement:** None but preferred
**Cut-Off time since graduation:** No limits set
**Program offers couple match:** Yes
**Visas Sponsored or accepted:** J1 visa

## Texas Health Presbyterian Hospital Dallas Internal Medicine Residency Program

**Specialty:** Internal Medicine
**Program name:** Texas Health Presbyterian Hospital Dallas Program
**Program code:** 140-48-11-420
**NRMP Code:** 1719140C0, 1719140P0
**Program type:** Community-based
**State:** Texas
**Address:** Presbyterian Hospital of Dallas, Department of Internal Medicine
        8200 Walnut Hill Ln, Dallas, TX  75231-4496
**Phone:** (214) 345-6176
**Fax:** (214) 345-5167
**Percentage of IMGs in the program:** 20%
**Minimum USMLE Step 1 Score Requirement:** 222
**Minimum USMLE Step 2 Score Requirement:** 222

**Attempts on any step:** Must pass on first attempt
**CS required at time of application:** Yes including ECFMG certificate
**USCE Requirement:** None
**Cut-Off time since graduation:** 3 years
**Program offers couple match:** Yes
**Visas Sponsored or accepted:** J1 visa


## Texas Tech University Health Sciences Center Paul L Foster School of Medicine Internal Medicine Residency Program

**Specialty:** Internal Medicine
**Program name:** Texas Tech University Health Sciences Center Paul L Foster School of Medicine Program
**Program code:** 140-48-11-424
**NRMP Code:** 1710140C1, 1710140C0
**Program type:** University-based
**State:** Texas
**Address:** Texas Tech University HSC Paul L Foster School of Medicine
          Internal Medicine Program, 4800 Alberta Ave, El Paso, TX 79905
**Phone:** (915) 545-6626    Ext: 252
**Fax:** (915) 545-6634
**Percentage of IMGs in the program:** 70%
**Minimum USMLE Step 1 Score Requirement:**

No limits set
**Minimum USMLE Step 2 Score Requirement:**
No limits set
**Attempts on any step:** No limits set
**CS required at time of application:** No, must
take by November
**USCE Requirement:** None
**Cut-Off time since graduation:** 10 years
**Program offers couple match:** Yes
**Visas Sponsored or accepted:** No visa

## University of Texas Southwestern Medical School (Austin) Internal Medicine Residency Program

**Specialty:** Internal Medicine
**Program name:** University of Texas
Southwestern Medical School (Austin) Program
**Program code:** 140-48-12-415
**NRMP Code:** 2835140P4, 2835140C2,
2835140P5
**Program type:** Community-based university
affiliated hospital
**State:** Texas
**Address:** University Medical Center at
Brackenridge, Department of Internal Medicine
        601 E 15th St, Austin, TX  78701
**Phone:** (512) 324-8355
**Fax:** (512) 324-8021
**Percentage of IMGs in the program:** 30%

**Minimum USMLE Step 1 Score Requirement:** 210
**Minimum USMLE Step 2 Score Requirement:** 210
**Attempts on any step:** Must pass on first attempt
**CS required at time of application:** Yes including ECFMG certificate
**USCE Requirement:** Yes, 1 month
**Cut-Off time since graduation:** 5 years
**Program offers couple match:** Yes
**Visas Sponsored or accepted:** J1 visa

## Methodist Health System Dallas Internal Medicine Residency Program

**Specialty:** Internal Medicine
**Program name:** Methodist Health System Dallas Program
**Program code:** 140-48-12-417
**NRMP Code:** 1707140C0
**Program type:** Community-based
**State:** Texas
**Address:** Methodist Hospital Dallas, GME Office
        1441 N Beckley Ave, Dallas, TX  75203-1201
**Phone:** (214) 947-2306
**Fax:** (214) 947-2306
**Percentage of IMGs in the program:** 20%

**Minimum USMLE Step 1 Score Requirement:** No limits set
**Minimum USMLE Step 2 Score Requirement:** No limits set
**Attempts on any step:** Must pass on first attempt
**CS required at time of application:** Yes including ECFMG certificate
**USCE Requirement:** None
**Cut-Off time since graduation:** 3 years
**Program offers couple match:** Yes
**Visas Sponsored or accepted:** J1 visa

## Methodist Hospital (Houston) Internal Medicine Residency Program

**Specialty:** Internal Medicine
**Program name:** Methodist Hospital (Houston) Program
**Program code:** 140-48-13-534
**NRMP Code:** 1167140C0
**Program type:** Community-based university affiliated hospital
**State:** Texas
**Address:** Methodist Hospital Houston, Smith Tower 1001
        6550 Fannin St, Houston, TX  77030
**Phone:** (713) 441-6729

**Fax:** (713) 790-6615
**Percentage of IMGs in the program:** 40%
**Minimum USMLE Step 1 Score Requirement:** 210
**Minimum USMLE Step 2 Score Requirement:** 210
**Attempts on any step:** Must pass on first attempt
**CS required at time of application:** No
**USCE Requirement:** None
**Cut-Off time since graduation:** 5 years
**Program offers couple match:** Yes
**Visas Sponsored or accepted:** J1 visa

## University of Texas Southwestern Medical School Internal Medicine Residency Program

**Specialty:** Internal Medicine
**Program name:** University of Texas Southwestern Medical School Program
**Program code:** 140-48-21-419
**NRMP Code:** 2835140P0, 2835140C0
**Program type:** University-based
**State:** Texas
**Address:** University of Texas Southwestern Medical Center
        Department of Medicine Education Office F5310B
        5323 Harry Hines Blvd, Dallas, TX

75390-9030
**Phone:** (214) 648-2287
**Fax:** (214) 648-7550
**Percentage of IMGs in the program:** 10%
**Minimum USMLE Step 1 Score Requirement:** 205
**Minimum USMLE Step 2 Score Requirement:** 205
**Attempts on any step:** No limits set
**CS required at time of application:** No
**USCE Requirement:** None
**Cut-Off time since graduation:** 5 years
**Program offers couple match:** Yes
**Visas Sponsored or accepted:** J1 visa

# University of Texas Medical Branch Hospitals Internal Medicine Residency Program

**Specialty:** Internal Medicine
**Program name:** University of Texas Medical Branch Hospitals Program
**Program code:** 140-48-21-421
**NRMP Code:** 1714140P3, 1714140C0, 1714140P0
**Program type:** University-based
**State:** Texas
**Address:** University of Texas Medical Branch Hospitals, Department of Internal Medicine
301 University Blvd, Galveston, TX

77555-0570
**Phone:** (409) 772-2653
**Fax:** (409) 772-5462
**Percentage of IMGs in the program:** 10% (Used to be 50% per year)
**Minimum USMLE Step 1 Score Requirement:** No limits set
**Minimum USMLE Step 2 Score Requirement:** No limits set
**Attempts on any step:** No limits set
**CS required at time of application:** No
**USCE Requirement:** None
**Cut-Off time since graduation:** 2 years
**Program offers couple match:** Yes
**Visas Sponsored or accepted:** J1 visa and H1b visa

## Baylor College of Medicine Internal Medicine Residency Program

**Specialty:** Internal Medicine
**Program name:** Baylor College of Medicine Program
**Program code:** 140-48-21-422
**NRMP Code:** 1716140C0, 1716140P0
**Program type:** University-based
**State:** Texas
**Address:** Baylor College of Medicine, Baylor Clinic Suite 1100-D

6620 Main St, Houston, TX  77030
**Phone:** (713) 798-0206
**Fax:** (713) 798-0223
**Percentage of IMGs in the program:** 0%
(Occasional 1 per year)
**Minimum USMLE Step 1 Score Requirement:**
230
**Minimum USMLE Step 2 Score Requirement:**
230
**Attempts on any step:** No limits set
**CS required at time of application:** No
**USCE Requirement:** None
**Cut-Off time since graduation:** 3 years
**Program offers couple match:** Yes
**Visas Sponsored or accepted:** J1 visa

# University of Texas Health Science Center at San Antonio Internal Medicine Residency Program

**Specialty:** Internal Medicine
**Program name:** University of Texas Health Science Center at San Antonio Program
**Program code:** 140-48-21-425
**NRMP Code:** 1722140C0, 1722140P1, 1722140P2, 1722140P0
**Program type:** University-based
**State:** Texas

**Address:** University of Texas HSC San Antonio, Office of Education MS 7871

7703 Floyd Curl Dr, San Antonio, TX 78229

**Phone:** (210) 567-6685
**Fax:** (210) 567-1739
**Percentage of IMGs in the program:** 15%
**Minimum USMLE Step 1 Score Requirement:** No limits set
**Minimum USMLE Step 2 Score Requirement:** No limits set
**Attempts on any step:** No limits set
**CS required at time of application:** Yes including ECFMG certificate
**USCE Requirement:** None
**Cut-Off time since graduation:** No limits set
**Program offers couple match:** Yes
**Visas Sponsored or accepted:** J1 visa

# Texas A&M College of Medicine-Scott and White Internal Medicine Residency Program

**Specialty:** Internal Medicine
**Program name:** Texas A&M College of Medicine-Scott and White Program
**Program code:** 140-48-21-426
**NRMP Code:** 1725140P0, 1725140C0
**Program type:** University-based

**State:** Texas
**Address:** Scott and White Memorial Hospital,
Graduate Medical Education,
      2401 S 31st St, Temple, TX 76508-0001
**Phone:** (254) 724-2364   Ext: 2364
**Fax:** (254) 724-4079
**Percentage of IMGs in the program:** 0%
(Occasional one)
**Minimum USMLE Step 1 Score Requirement:**
225
**Minimum USMLE Step 2 Score Requirement:**
225
**Attempts on any step:** No limits set
**CS required at time of application:** Yes
including ECFMG certificate
**USCE Requirement:** None
**Cut-Off time since graduation:** 3 years
**Program offers couple match:** Yes
**Visas Sponsored or accepted:** J1 visa

# Texas Tech University (Lubbock) Internal Medicine Residency Program

Specialty: Internal Medicine
Program name: Texas Tech University (Lubbock)
Program
Program code: 140-48-21-459
**NRMP Code:** 2973140P0, 2973140C0
**Program type:** University-based

**State:** Texas
**Address:** Texas Tech University HSC Lubbock,
Department of Medicine MS 9410,
          3601 4th St, Lubbock, TX  79430
**Phone:** (806) 743-3155    Ext:  237
**Fax:** (806) 743-3143
**Percentage of IMGs in the program:** 60%
**Minimum USMLE Step 1 Score Requirement:**
No limits set
**Minimum USMLE Step 2 Score Requirement:**
No limits set
**Attempts on any step:** No limits set
**CS required at time of application:** Yes
including ECFMG certificate
**USCE Requirement:** None
**Cut-Off time since graduation:** 7 years
**Program offers couple match:** Yes
**Visas Sponsored or accepted:** J1 visa


## Texas Tech University (Amarillo) Internal Medicine Residency Program


**Specialty:** Internal Medicine
**Program name:** Texas Tech University
(Amarillo) Program
**Program code:** 140-48-21-477
**NRMP Code:** 2993140C0
**Program type:** Community-based university

affiliated hospital
**State:** Texas
**Address:** Texas Tech University HSC Amarillo,
Internal Medicine Program,
          1400 Coulter Rd, Amarillo, TX  79106
**Phone:** (806) 354-5489
**Fax:** (806) 354-5765
**Percentage of IMGs in the program:** 90%
**Minimum USMLE Step 1 Score Requirement:**
220
**Minimum USMLE Step 2 Score Requirement:**
220
**Attempts on any step:** Must pass on first
attempt including CS exam
**CS required at time of application:** Yes
including ECFMG certificate
**USCE Requirement:** None
**Cut-Off time since graduation:** No limits set
**Program offers couple match:** Yes
**Visas Sponsored or accepted:** J1 visa (limited
number)

# Texas Tech University (Permian Basin) Internal Medicine Residency Program

**Specialty:** Internal Medicine
**Program name:** Texas Tech University (Permian
Basin) Program
**Program code:** 140-48-21-519

**NRMP Code:** 3124140C0
**Program type:** University-based
**State:** Texas
**Address:** Texas Tech University HSC Odessa, Internal Medicine Program,
            701 W 5th St, Odessa, TX  79763
**Phone:** (432) 703-5340
**Fax:** (432) 335-5297
**Percentage of IMGs in the program:** 70%
**Minimum USMLE Step 1 Score Requirement:** 220
**Minimum USMLE Step 2 Score Requirement:** 220
**Attempts on any step:** Must pass maximum on the 3rd attempt
**CS required at time of application:** Yes including ECFMG certificate
**USCE Requirement:** None
**Cut-Off time since graduation:** No limits set but prefer 5 years
**Program offers couple match:** Yes
**Visas Sponsored or accepted:** J1 visa


# University of Texas Health Science Center at San Antonio Lower Rio Grande Valley RAHC Internal Medicine Residency Program


**Specialty:** Internal Medicine

**Program name:** University of Texas Health Science Center at San Antonio Lower Rio Grande Valley RAHC Program
**Program code:** 140-48-21-524
**NRMP Code:** 1722140C1
**Program type:** Community-based university affiliated hospital
**State:** Texas
**Address:** Rio Grande Valley Reg Academic Health Center, Room 213603,
          2102 Treasure Hills Blvd, Harlingen, TX 78550
**Phone:** (956) 365-8805
**Fax:** (956) 389-4603
**Percentage of IMGs in the program:** 80%
**Minimum USMLE Step 1 Score Requirement:** No limits set
**Minimum USMLE Step 2 Score Requirement:** No limits set
**Attempts on any step:** Must pass on first attempt
**CS required at time of application:** No
**USCE Requirement:** Yes, at least 1 month
**Cut-Off time since graduation:** No limits set
**Program offers couple match:** Yes
**Visas Sponsored or accepted:** J1 visa

# University of Texas at Houston Internal Medicine Residency Program

**Specialty:** Internal Medicine
**Program name:** University of Texas at Houston Program
**Program code:** 140-48-31-423
**NRMP Code:** 2923140C0, 2923140P0, 2923140P1
**Program type:** University-based
**State:** Texas
**Address:** University of Texas Medical School at Houston,

Department of Internal Medicine Suite 134,

6431 Fannin St, Houston, TX  77030
**Phone:** (713) 500-6536
**Fax:** (713) 500-6530
**Percentage of IMGs in the program:** 40%
**Minimum USMLE Step 1 Score Requirement:** No limits set
**Minimum USMLE Step 2 Score Requirement:** No limits set
**Attempts on any step:** Must pass on first attempt
**CS required at time of application:** Yes including ECFMG certificate
**USCE Requirement:** Yes, 3 months
**Cut-Off time since graduation:** No limits set

**Program offers couple match:** Yes
**Visas Sponsored or accepted:** J1 visa

# Utah

## University of Utah Internal Medicine Residency Program

**Specialty:** Internal Medicine
**Program name:** University of Utah Program
**Program code:** 140-49-21-427
**NRMP Code:** 1732140P0, 1732140P1, 1732140C0, 1732140C1, 1732140C2
**Program type:** University-based
**State:** Utah
**Address:** University of Utah Medical Center, Department of Internal Medical Room 4C116
          30 N 1900 E, Salt Lake City, UT  84132
**Phone:** (801) 581-7899
**Fax:** (801) 585-0418
**Percentage of IMGs in the program:** 10%
**Minimum USMLE Step 1 Score Requirement:** 230
**Minimum USMLE Step 2 Score Requirement:** 230
**Attempts on any step:** Must pass on first attempt

**CS required at time of application:** Yes
including ECFMG certificate
**USCE Requirement:** None
**Cut-Off time since graduation:** 5 years
**Program offers couple match:** Yes
**Visas Sponsored or accepted:** J1 visa

# Vermont

## University of Vermont/Fletcher Allen Health Care Internal Medicine Residency Program

**Specialty:** Internal Medicine
**Program name:** University of Vermont/Fletcher Allen Health Care Program
**Program code:** 140-50-21-429
**NRMP Code:** 1734140P0, 1734140M0, 1734140C0, 1734140P2
**Program type:** University-based
**State:** Vermont
**Address:** University of Vermont FAHC, Smith 244
          111 Colchester Ave, Burlington, VT 05401
**Phone:** (802) 847-4953
**Percentage of IMGs in the program:** 7%

**Minimum USMLE Step 1 Score Requirement:** No limits set
**Minimum USMLE Step 2 Score Requirement:** No limits set
**Attempts on any step:** Must pass on first attempt
**CS required at time of application:** Yes including ECFMG certificate
**USCE Requirement:** Yes, at least 1 month
**Cut-Off time since graduation:** 2 years
**Program offers couple match:** Yes
**Visas Sponsored or accepted:** J1 visa

# Virginia

## University of Virginia Internal Medicine Residency Program

**Specialty:** Internal Medicine
**Program name:** University of Virginia Program
**Program code:** 140-51-21-430
**Program type:** University-based
**State:** Virginia
**Address:** University of Virginia Health System, Department of Medicine
          PO Box 800466, Charlottesville, VA 22908
**Phone:** (434) 924-2408

**Fax:** (434) 243-0399
**Percentage of IMGs in the program:** 5% (Not yearly)
**Minimum USMLE Step 1 Score Requirement:** 210
**Minimum USMLE Step 2 Score Requirement:** 210
**Attempts on any step:** Must pass on first attempt
**CS required at time of application:** Yes including ECFMG certificate
**USCE Requirement:** Yes, 1 year
**Cut-Off time since graduation:** 5 years
**Program offers couple match:** Yes
**Visas Sponsored or accepted:** J1 visa

## Eastern Virginia Medical School Internal Medicine Residency Program

**Specialty:** Internal Medicine
**Program name:** Eastern Virginia Medical School Program
**Program code:** 140-51-21-432
**NRMP Code:** 2980140P0, 2980140C1, 2980140C0
**Program type:** Community-based
**State:** Virginia
**Address:** Eastern Virginia Medical School,

Hofheimer Hall Suite 410
          825 Fairfax Ave, Norfolk, VA  23507
**Phone:** (757) 446-5794
**Fax:** (757) 446-7921
**Percentage of IMGs in the program:** 40%
**Minimum USMLE Step 1 Score Requirement:**
225
**Minimum USMLE Step 2 Score Requirement:**
225
**Attempts on any step:** Must pass on first
attempt
**CS required at time of application:** Yes
including ECFMG certificate
**USCE Requirement:** Yes, 1 year
**Cut-Off time since graduation:** 5 yeas
**Program offers couple match:** Yes
**Visas Sponsored or accepted:** J1 visa


## Virginia Commonwealth University Health System Internal Medicine Residency Program

**Specialty:** Internal Medicine
**Program name:** Virginia Commonwealth
University Health System Program
**Program code:** 140-51-21-433
**NRMP Code:** 1743140C0, 1743140P0,
1743140P1, 1743140P2
**Program type:** University-based

**State:** Virginia
**Address:** VCU Health System, PO Box 980509
　　　　　1200 E Broad St, Richmond, VA
23298-0509
**Phone:** (804) 828-9726
**Fax:** (804) 828-4926
**Percentage of IMGs in the program:** 3%
**Minimum USMLE Step 1 Score Requirement:**
No limits set
**Minimum USMLE Step 2 Score Requirement:**
No limits set
**Attempts on any step:** No limits set
**CS required at time of application:** No
**USCE Requirement:** Yes, 3 months
**Cut-Off time since graduation:** 4 years
**Program offers couple match:** Yes
**Visas Sponsored or accepted:** J1 visa

## Carilion Clinic-Virginia Tech Carilion School of Medicine Internal Medicine Residency Program

**Specialty:** Internal Medicine
**Program name:** Carilion Clinic-Virginia Tech
Carilion School of Medicine Program
**Program code:** 140-51-31-431
**NRMP Code:** 1748140C0, 1748140P0
**Program type:** Community-based university
affiliated hospital

**State:** Virginia
**Address:** Carilion Clinic, Department of Medicine PO Box 13367
          1906 Belleview Ave, Roanoke, VA 24014
**Phone:** (540) 981-7120
**Percentage of IMGs in the program:** 40%
**Minimum USMLE Step 1 Score Requirement:** 210
**Minimum USMLE Step 2 Score Requirement:** 210
**Attempts on any step:** Must pass on first attempt
**CS required at time of application:** Yes including ECFMG certificate
**USCE Requirement:** Yes, 6 months
**Cut-Off time since graduation:** 5 years
**Program offers couple match:** Yes
**Visas Sponsored or accepted:** J1 visa

# Washington

## Providence Sacred Heart Medical Center (Spokane) Internal Medicine Residency Program

**Specialty:** Internal Medicine

**Program name:** Providence Sacred Heart Medical Center (Spokane) Program
**Program code:** 140-54-31-436
**NRMP Code:** 1758140C0
**Program type:** Community-based university affiliated hospital
**State:** Washington
**Address:** Providence Sacred Heart Medical Center, Internal Medicine Program
       101 W 8th Ave, Spokane, WA  99220
**Phone:** (509) 474-3237
**Fax:** (509) 474-5316
**Percentage of IMGs in the program:** 25%
**Minimum USMLE Step 1 Score Requirement:** 210
**Minimum USMLE Step 2 Score Requirement:** 210
**Attempts on any step:** Must pass on first attempt
**CS required at time of application:** No
**USCE Requirement:** Yes 2 months
**Cut-Off time since graduation:** 5 years
**Program offers couple match:** Yes
**Visas Sponsored or accepted:** No visa

# West Virginia

## Marshall University School of Medicine Internal Medicine Residency Program

**Specialty:** Internal Medicine
**Program name:** Marshall University School of Medicine Program
**Program code:** 140-55-21-439
**State:** West Virginia
**Address:** Marshall University School of Medicine, Department of Medicine,
        1249 15th St, Huntington, WV  25701-3655
**Phone:** (304) 691-1086
**Fax:** (304) 691-1693
**Percentage of IMGs in the program:** 70%
**Minimum USMLE Step 1 Score Requirement:** 225
**Minimum USMLE Step 2 Score Requirement:** 225
**Attempts on any step:** No limits set
**CS required at time of application:** Yes including ECFMG certificate
**USCE Requirement:** None
**Cut-Off time since graduation:** 5 years
**Program offers couple match:** Yes
**Visas Sponsored or accepted:** J1 visa

# West Virginia University Internal Medicine Residency Program

**Specialty:** Internal Medicine
**Program name:** West Virginia University Program
**Program code:** 140-55-11-440
**NRMP Code:** 1837140C0
**Program type:** University-based
**State:** West Virginia
**Address:** West Virginia University HSC, RCB Health Sciences Center Box 9168
One Medical Center Dr, Morgantown, WV  26506-9168
**Phone:** (304) 293-4239
**Fax:** (304) 293-3651
**Percentage of IMGs in the program:** 20%
**Minimum USMLE Step 1 Score Requirement:** No limits set
**Minimum USMLE Step 2 Score Requirement:** No limits set
**Attempts on any step:** No limits set, but prefer those with no attempts
**CS required at time of application:** Yes including ECFMG certificate
**USCE Requirement:** None but 3 months is highly preferred
**Cut-Off time since graduation:** 4 years
**Program offers couple match:** Yes
**Visas Sponsored or accepted:** J1 visa

## Charleston Area Medical Center/West Virginia University (Charleston Division) Internal Medicine Residency Program

**Specialty:** Internal Medicine
**Program name:** Charleston Area Medical Center/West Virginia University (Charleston Division) Program
**Program code:** 140-55-11-438
**NRMP Code:** 1902140C0, 1902140P0
**Program type:** Community-based university affiliated hospital
**State:** West Virginia
**Address:** Charleston Area Medical Center, Department of Internal Medicine
3110 MacCorkle Ave SE, Charleston, WV  25304
**Phone:** (304) 347-1341
**Fax:** (304) 347-1344
**Percentage of IMGs in the program:** 60%
**Minimum USMLE Step 1 Score Requirement:** 220
**Minimum USMLE Step 2 Score Requirement:** 220
**Attempts on any step:** Must pass from maximum the second attempt on any step

**CS required at time of application:** Yes including ECFMG certificate
**USCE Requirement:** Yes
**Cut-Off time since graduation:** No limits set
**Program offers couple match:** Yes
**Visas Sponsored or accepted:** J1 visa

## Wisconsin

### Gundersen Lutheran Medical Foundation Internal Medicine Program

**Specialty:** Internal Medicine
**Program name:** Gundersen Lutheran Medical Foundation Program
**Program code:** 140-56-12-442
**NRMP Code:** 1774140C0
**Program type:** Community-based
**State:** Wisconsin
**Address:** Gundersen Lutheran Medical Foundation, C03-006A
        1836 South Ave, La Crosse, WI  54601-5429
**Phone:** (608) 775-2923
**Fax:** (608) 775-1548
**Percentage of IMGs in the program:** 30%

**Minimum USMLE Step 1 Score Requirement:** No limits set
**Minimum USMLE Step 2 Score Requirement:** No limits set
**Attempts on any step:** Must pass on first attempt
**CS required at time of application:** Yes including ECFMG certificate
**USCE Requirement:** None
**Cut-Off time since graduation:** 2 years
**Program offers couple match:** Yes
**Visas Sponsored or accepted:** J1 visa and H1b visa

## University of Wisconsin Internal Medicine Residency Program

**Specialty:** Internal Medicine
**Program name:** University of Wisconsin Program
**Program code:** 140-56-21-443
**NRMP Code:** 1779140C0, 1779140M0,
**Program type:** University-based
**State:** Wisconsin
**Address:** University of Wisconsin Hospital and Clinics, Suite 5000 Centenniel Building
        1685 Highland Ave, Madison, WI 53792
**Phone:** (608) 263-7350

**Fax:** (608) 262-6743
**Percentage of IMGs in the program:** 8%
**Minimum USMLE Step 1 Score Requirement:** No limits set
**Minimum USMLE Step 2 Score Requirement:** No limits set
**Attempts on any step:** Maximum of 3 attempts
**CS required at time of application:** No
**USCE Requirement:** None
**Cut-Off time since graduation:** 10 years
**Program offers couple match:** Yes
**Visas Sponsored or accepted:** J1 visa

## Aurora Health Care Program

**Specialty:** Internal Medicine
**Program name:** Aurora Health Care Program
**Program code:** 140-56-21-446
**NRMP Code:** 1787140C0
**Program type:** Community-based university affiliated hospital
**State:** Wisconsin
**Address:** Aurora Sinai Medical Center, PO Box 342

       945 N 12th St, Milwaukee, WI  53201-0342
**Phone:** (414) 219-7635
**Fax:** (414) 219-4539
**Percentage of IMGs in the program:** 40%
**Minimum USMLE Step 1 Score Requirement:** 211

**Minimum USMLE Step 2 Score Requirement:** 211
**Attempts on any step:** Must pass on first attempt
**CS required at time of application:** Yes including ECFMG certificate
**USCE Requirement:** None
**Cut-Off time since graduation:** No limits set
**Program offers couple match:** Yes
**Visas Sponsored or accepted:** No visa

## Marshfield Clinic-St Joseph's Hospital Internal Medicine Residency Program

**Specialty:** Internal Medicine
**Program name:** Marshfield Clinic-St Joseph's Hospital Program
**Program code:** 140-56-31-444
**NRMP Code:** 1780140C0
**Program type:** Community-based university affiliated hospital
**State:** Wisconsin
**Address:** Marshfield Clinic, Department of Internal Med 3K2
        1000 N Oak Ave, Marshfield, WI  54449
**Phone:** (715) 387-5260
**Fax:** (715) 387-5434
**Percentage of IMGs in the program:** 30%

**Minimum USMLE Step 1 Score Requirement:** 210
**Minimum USMLE Step 2 Score Requirement:** 210
**Attempts on any step:** Must pass maximum on 2nd attempt on any step
**CS required at time of application:** Yes including ECFMG certificate
**USCE Requirement:** Yes, 4 months
**Cut-Off time since graduation:** 5 years unless had good scores and recent USCE or residency
**Program offers couple match:** Yes
**Visas Sponsored or accepted:** J1 visa and H1b visa

## Medical College of Wisconsin Affiliated Hospitals Internal Medicine Residency Program

**Specialty:** Internal Medicine
**Program name:** Medical College of Wisconsin Affiliated Hospitals Program
**Program code:** 140-56-31-445
**NRMP Code:** 1784140C2, 1784140C0, 1784140C1, 1784140M0, 1784140P0
**Program type:** University-based
**State:** Wisconsin
**Address:** Medical College of Wisconsin, Department of Medicine CLCC C5119
            9200 W Wisconsin Ave, Milwaukee,

WI 53226
**Phone:** (414) 805-0532
**Fax:** (414) 805-0535
**Percentage of IMGs in the program:** 0%
(Occasional one)
**Minimum USMLE Step 1 Score Requirement:**
220
**Minimum USMLE Step 2 Score Requirement:**
220
**Attempts on any step:** Must pass on the first
attempt including CS exam
**CS required at time of application:** Yes
including ECFMG certificate
**USCE Requirement:** Yes, 3 months
**Cut-Off time since graduation:** 3 years
**Program offers couple match:** Yes
**Visas Sponsored or accepted:** J1 visa

**Please take 1 minute to write a review and rate our book on Amazon. We wish you a successful match. Thank you for buying our book.**

If you have any questions please email us at applicantguide@yahoo.com

**IMG Guide**
**&**
**Applicant Guide**

www.imgguide.com
www.applicantguide.com